Financial Information, Resources, Services, and Tools (FIRST)

Education Debt Manager

for Matriculating and Graduating Medical School Students

FIRST is a program of the AAMC
aamc.org/FIRST

The AAMC (Association of American Medical Colleges) is a nonprofit association dedicated to improving the health of people everywhere through medical education, health care, medical research, and community collaborations. Its members comprise all 155 accredited U.S. and 16 accredited Canadian medical schools; approximately 400 teaching hospitals and health systems, including Department of Veterans Affairs medical centers; and more than 70 academic societies. Through these institutions and organizations, the AAMC leads and serves America's medical schools and teaching hospitals and the millions of individuals employed across academic medicine, including more than 191,000 full-time faculty members, 95,000 medical students, 149,000 resident physicians, and 60,000 graduate students and postdoctoral researchers in the biomedical sciences. In 2022, the Association of Academic Health Centers and the Association of Academic Health Centers International merged into the AAMC, broadening the AAMC's U.S. membership and expanding its reach to international academic health centers. Learn more at aamc.org.

Information within the *Education Debt Manager* is based on AAMC estimates and interpretation of federal regulations effective January 2022. Information is subject to change based on changes in federal regulations and/or at the discretion of the secretary of the Department of Education. For exact loan balances and information on repayment, students and graduates should contact the servicers of their student loans.

Please note: AAMC-published materials are intended to provide general information and are not intended to fulfill or replace any federally mandated requirements.

Published August 2022.

ISBN: 978-1-57754-207-0

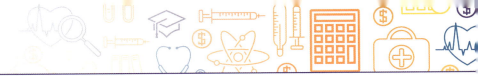

A Note From FIRST

Congratulations! Whether you are beginning or completing your medical education, you have worked hard to get to where you are today, and the purpose of this publication is to help you develop a strategy for the successful management of your education debt. Most of the repayment options and programs discussed are applicable only to federal student loans — the type of debt that is the bulk (if not all) of what is borrowed by medical students.

Managing student loans may seem like a daunting, confusing, and sometimes downright frustrating task. Despite this, it is vital to your financial future that you clearly understand the financial decisions you will make in the immediate future and that you equip yourself with the knowledge to choose the best option possible.

This resource, the *Education Debt Manager*, is designed to help students, residents, and financial aid staff navigate the complexities of medical student debt. Not only will this information help you borrow monies strategically, it will also enable you to make wise repayment decisions by enhancing your understanding of important debt management skills for future use (including during the lean years of residency).

Benjamin Franklin has been attributed with saying, "An investment in knowledge always pays the best interest." Be encouraged and know that this major investment you are making in yourself, your future, and the future of health care will be rewarding, both personally and professionally.

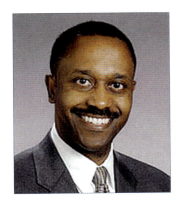

Gary LeRoy, MD
Associate Dean
Wright State University
Boonshoft School of Medicine

The best advice I received when I was contemplating a career in medicine was to concentrate my initial efforts on getting into medical school and leave the issue of how to pay for it for another day. Advisors assured me that there would be enough money available in the form of scholarships, grants, and low-interest loans to pay for my medical education.

What they did not educate me about was debt management, the principle of compound interest, and that it could take me the bulk of my professional career to pay off my student loans.

It has been more than 20 years since I heard those words of advice, and I've been passing them along to prospective medical students ever since. However, I qualify my comments today with the fact that the trend line for medical student indebtedness has become increasingly steep with each academic year.

Students must arrive at the door of the house of medicine with an enhanced awareness of how they will navigate the rising tide of medical education debt they will encounter prior to their graduation.

On April 6, 2022, the U.S. Department of Education extended COVID-19 emergency relief for student loans through Aug. 31, 2022. Relief measures for eligible loans include suspension of loan payments, 0% interest rate (March 13, 2020, through Aug. 31, 2022), and no collections on defaulted loans.

The numbers and values related to student loan costs presented in this publication reflect student loan emergency relief measures from March 13, 2020, to Jan. 31, 2022, and this publication will be updated again in spring 2023.

Visit the Federal Student Aid website for the most current information related to student loan emergency relief measures and your federal student loans: StudentAid.gov/coronavirus.

Contents

Education Debt

Paying for a medical education is challenging. In fact, the majority of medical school graduates complete their education with the assistance of student loan financing — primarily in the form of federal student loans. In the graduating class of 2021, 73% of medical students reported leaving medical school with student loan debt. Across the country, the median level of debt for the class of 2021 was $200,000, including undergraduate debt (based on surveys of students at public and private MD-granting medical schools).

The AAMC collects this type of data each year, and we share it with you as a point of reference. In the spring of your graduating year, immediately before leaving medical school, you will also be asked to share your feedback about your medical school experience via a survey called the Graduation Questionnaire (GQ).

We thank you in advance for taking the time to provide your valuable input on all aspects of your medical education; it helps improve medical education for future students. The information below is updated every year. The fact card for the class of 2022 will be available in October. To view the current information, visit aamc.org/first/debtfacts.

OCTOBER 2021
Medical Student Education:
Debt, Costs, and Loan Repayment
Fact Card for the Class of 2021

AAMC

Education Debt	Public	Private	All
Percentage with education debt	74%	70%	73%
Mean education debt of indebted only (versus 2020, %)	$194,280 (↓3%)	$218,746 (↓0.5%)	$203,062 (↓2%)
Median education debt of indebted only (versus 2020, %)	$195,000 (↓3%)	$220,000 (0%)	$200,000 (0%)

Education Debt (including premedical)	Percentage of Graduates		
	Public	Private	All
$100,000 or more	84%	82%	83%
$200,000 or more	49%	59%	53%
$300,000 or more	14%	27%	19%
Planning to enter loan forgiveness or repayment program			47%

Education Debt Breakdown	Percentage of Graduates	Median Debt
Premedical education debt	30%	$27,000
Medical education debt	69%	$200,000

Noneducation Debt	Percentage of Graduates	Median Debt
Credit cards	10%	$4,000
Residency and relocation loans	1%	$10,000

Source of data in tables above: FIRST analysis of AAMC 2021 Graduation Questionnaire data. Education debt figures include premedical education debt plus medical education debt.

Cost, In-State, 2021-22	Public	Private
Tuition and fees, first-year median	$40,562 (↑4%)	$65,650 (↑3%)
Cost of attendance (COA), first-year median	$65,085 (↑2%)	$90,138 (↑3%)
4-year COA for class of 2022, median	$263,488 (↑1%)	$357,868 (↑3%)

Source: AAMC TSF Survey data from 88 public schools and 57 private schools.

aamc.org/FIRST

Association of
American Medical Colleges

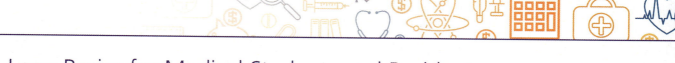

Loan Basics for Medical Students and Residents

Getting Organized

The first step in managing your education debt is getting organized. Once you have all your documents gathered and organized in a single place, you will be better prepared to manage your debt.

MedLoans® Organizer and Calculator

When putting your essential documents in order, you may rely on a folder system, a filing cabinet, a scanning-and-saving process, or even a shoebox. The specific method you use is not as important as the actual process of opening, reading — yes, reading — and saving your student loan documents.

To help you stay organized during medical school and residency, the AAMC has created an online resource specifically designed for medical students and residents to safely and securely organize and save loan portfolio information as well as calculate various repayment options. This tool can help you understand the impact of your borrowing (that is, total interest cost) before you even accept a loan disbursement and provide total estimated costs for different repayment strategies. Use the MedLoans Organizer and Calculator as you borrow and manage these loans throughout repayment — it will empower you to make educated decisions about your student loans.

Use your AAMC username and password to log in to the MedLoans Organizer and Calculator.

aamc.org/medloans

For help with your username and password, contact Denine Hales at dhales@aamc.org.

To quickly and easily use the MedLoans Organizer and Calculator, log in to your Federal Student Aid (FSA) account and select "Download My Aid Data" at the top of the page. The downloaded file with your loan information can then be uploaded directly into your MedLoans Organizer. Just a few simple steps allow you to see estimates based solely on your debt situation and potential career path. (The next page has more information.)

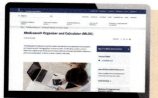

- Upload your student loan data (details on page 7).
- Keep track of your student loan information.
- Develop personalized repayment strategies.

> "Loans are less scary, and I've made a strategy to confront them. I'm also more confident that I can manage my debt during residency and beyond after using the MedLoans Calculator."

Nathaniel Bayer
University of Rochester School
of Medicine and Dentistry

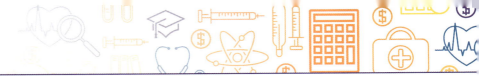

Know the Details of Your Loans

The next step to managing education debt is knowing the details of your loan portfolio — including the types of loans you borrowed, the dates of disbursement, and the name of the servicer that you will eventually send payments to. Good records will help you transition more easily into successful student loan management when that time comes. However, if you do not have all of your loan information now, don't despair. There are two resources you can rely on to find the details of your debt:

- The financial aid office (premed and medical) may be able to help you identify the details of the loans borrowed.

- Your Federal Student Aid (FSA) account is where you will find details on your federal student loans. Visit StudentAid.gov.

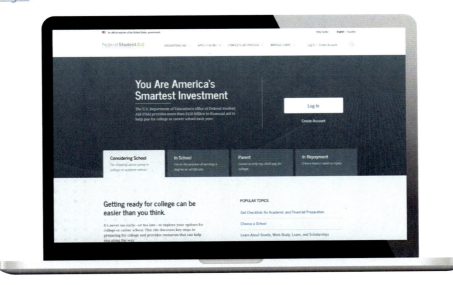

StudentAid.gov

To log in, provide your username and password.

If you do not have a Federal Student Aid (FSA) ID, you will select the "Create an FSA ID" tab.

Most of the repayment options and programs discussed in the following sections are applicable to federal student loans only. Inside your FSA account are details for most of your federal loans, including the current lender, servicer, and outstanding principal balance (OPB) of each loan. This information is not real-time data, and due to processing times and only periodic updates, your current loan balance may be different from what you see in your FSA account. For the most up-to-date information, contact your loan servicers.

The only federal loans that will not be displayed in your FSA account are Loans for Disadvantaged Students (LDS) and Primary Care Loans (PCL). **Nonfederal loans (including private and institutional loans) are also not listed in your FSA account.**

To find the details of loans not shown in your FSA account, consult with your financial aid office or review your credit report (annualcreditreport.com).

Lenders

To finance their education, most medical students borrow federally guaranteed student loans from the Direct Loan (DL) program, also known as the **William D. Ford Federal Direct Loan** program (StudentAid.gov).

Currently, the DL program is the only lender disbursing federal student loans. The DL program lends money to borrowers directly from the U.S. Department of Education, including Direct Unsubsidized Loans, Direct PLUS Loans, and Direct Consolidation Loans.

Perkins Loans, Primary Care Loans (PCL), and Loans for Disadvantaged Students (LDS) are also federal student loans. However, these loans are issued by a school on behalf of the federal government.

Once you know who your lenders are, the next and more important step is to find out who services the loans. The loan servicer is important because, after separating from school, and until loans are fully repaid, **the servicer will be your point of contact for everything concerning these loans.**

Servicers

After a lender disburses the loan, a servicer oversees the administration of the loan. Servicers also handle most activities that occur during repayment, such as making payments, updating your contact information, processing requests to postpone payments, and providing tax forms for potential student loan interest deductions. The servicers of your loans can change. To stay informed about these changes, be sure to open and read all communications you receive about your student loans, and if you have questions, call the loan servicer immediately.

For successful loan repayment, it's crucial that you know the servicers of your loans and how to contact them. To find the loan servicer for each of your federal student loans, log in to your FSA account at StudentAid.gov.

Private Loans

The cost of your medical education, including all living expenses, should be completely covered by your financial aid package (consisting of federal and institutional loans). If all of your expenses are not covered, you may look at private loans to supplement your financial situation.

Private education loans may be less favorable than federal debt for a variety of reasons, including lack of forgiveness programs, limited postponement options, and reduced control over the actual amount of the required monthly payment.

The discrepancy between federal and private student loans exists because private education debt is not regulated by the legislation that governs federal student loans, meaning the terms and conditions of private loans are at the discretion of the private lender. Most of the repayment options and programs discussed in this document are applicable only to your federal student loans.

Students Needing Additional Funds

Borrowing private loans should be done only after careful consideration. If you find yourself in need of additional funds during medical school, visit your financial aid office to discuss other possible options.

If private education loans are already a part of your debt portfolio, you'll want to reach out to the private lender to determine the terms and conditions that exist on those loans in order to better know how to manage them.

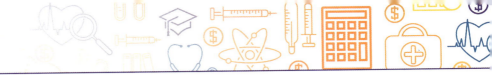

Resolving Disputes

If you are dissatisfied with your experience in the federal student aid process, you can file a formal complaint at the FSA Feedback Center. However, if your situation involves a disagreement with a loan servicer, prior to submitting a complaint, you are encouraged to first work directly with your loan servicer to seek a resolution.

If a resolution cannot be found, then submitting a formal complaint, at the FSA Feedback Center, is warranted. Once a complaint is received, the U.S. Department of Education's FSA office works to provide resolution within 60 days (if applicable and pending the availability of all necessary data).

Reasons to Contact Your Loan Servicer

- You have questions about your loans.
- You want to make voluntary payments.
- You need help selecting an affordable repayment plan.
- You changed your name, address, or phone number.
- You dropped below half-time enrollment or take a leave of absence (LOA).
- You've graduated from medical school.
- You want to select or change repayment plans.

Ombudsman Group

If you disagree with the response provided to your complaint, or believe it to be incorrect, you can contact the Federal Student Aid Ombudsman Group for additional assistance in gaining resolution. The Ombudsman Group is a neutral and confidential resource that aids in resolving disputes about federal student loans. Though, realize, it does not take "sides," does not have the power to make binding decisions, and cannot overturn decisions of other entities. The Ombudsman Group can be reached at StudentAid.gov/ombudsman or 1-877-557-2575.

Resources for Borrowers

If you experience problems or disputes with your loans, several resources are available to assist you, including:

FSA Feedback Center (for issues involving federal student loans)
1-844-651-0077 • StudentAid.gov/feedback

U.S. Department of Education FSA Ombudsman Group
1-877-557-2575 • StudentAid.gov/ombudsman

Student Loan Borrower Assistance Project
studentloanborrowerassistance.org

Consumer Financial Protection Bureau (for issues involving private student loans)
1-855-411-2372 • consumerfinance.gov

Debt Resolution for Defaulted Federal Student Aid
myeddebt.ed.gov

Total and Permanent Disability (TPD) Discharge Application
secure.disabilitydischarge.com/registration

Master Promissory Note (MPN)

The Master Promissory Note (MPN) is a legally binding contract between you and the lender of your federal student loans (the U.S. Department of Education). Simply stated, an MPN is your documented promise to repay the debt under the specified terms. The Department of Education's Informed Borrowing Confirmation process allows you to complete the Annual Student Loan Acknowledgment (ASLA) by logging in to your Federal Student Aid account at StudentAid.gov. This acknowledgment confirms that you are aware of your outstanding level of debt before you receive additional Direct Loans.

The obligation to repay your student loan debt is a serious responsibility that cannot be excused, even if:

- Your course of study is not completed (or not completed in the regular amount of time).
- You do not receive the education program or service that you purchased.
- You are unable to obtain employment.
- You are dissatisfied with your education experience.

Rights	Responsibilities
• Prepay any federal loan without penalty.	• Complete exit counseling before leaving or dropping below half-time enrollment.
• Request a copy of your MPN.	• Make loan payments on time.
• Change repayment plans.	• Make payments despite nonreceipt of a bill.
• Receive grace periods and subsidies on certain loans.	• Notify the servicers of changes to your contact or personal information.
• Use deferment or forbearance to postpone payments.	• Notify the servicers of changes in your enrollment status.
• Receive documentation of loan obligations, rights and responsibilities, and when the loan is fully repaid.	

For a complete list of a borrower's rights and responsibilities, review the Borrower's Rights and Responsibilities Statement located in the MPN. Questions about this list or the terms and conditions of your federal student loans can be directed to the lender, servicer, or your medical school's financial aid office.

Less Than Full-Time, Leave of Absence, and Withdrawing

During medical school, if your status changes due to course load or enrollment dropping below half-time, a leave of absence (LOA), or a withdrawal from the program, then loan repayment will begin on all your federal student loans. This means, if a loan has a grace period, it will begin the moment any of the scenarios above occur. In addition, if you're in one of these situations and return to full-time status after six or more months, any federal student loans qualifying for grace periods will no longer qualify for another grace period (e.g., upon graduation from medical school). Loan payments could be due on these loans immediately after graduating.

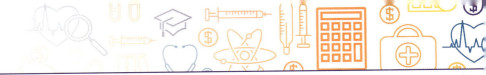

If your full-time status does change, it is critical that you contact the financial aid office staff immediately. They will:

1) Guide you through the required exit counseling for your loans.

2) Update you on which loans require immediate repayment and which ones have a grace period.

If you think you may have experienced a status change while you were enrolled but aren't sure if this resulted in using your grace period, you can contact your school's financial aid office or reach out to your loan servicers to see if your existing loans have a grace period and when repayment is currently scheduled to begin.

Delinquency and Default

Medical school borrowers have a very low default rate. This means that borrowers like you repay their loans and repay them on time, and many even pay them off earlier than required. The key to duplicating this positive repayment behavior with your debt portfolio is staying organized and knowing when your payments are due.

During medical school and residency, consider using automatic payment services such as online banking to schedule automatic student loan payments from your checking or savings account. Scheduling automatic payments can be used as a strategy to ensure that all reoccurring payments (loans, credit cards, utilities, etc.) are made on time.

Though payments are not required while one is enrolled in medical school, when the time comes to repay student loans, if something slips through the cracks, the loan will be considered delinquent on the first day that the payment is late. If a scheduled payment isn't made for 270 days, then the loan is considered in default.

There are negative consequences for both these situations (refer to the list above). Each will hurt your credit well into the future, causing problems if you need credit for a house, a practice, and many, if not all, other consumer loans.

The record of defaulted loans remains on a credit report for at least seven years. If you are experiencing financial difficulties, do not wait until it's too late — call your servicers to see what arrangements can be made.

Consequences of ...

Delinquency
- Credit bureaus are notified.
- Credit is negatively affected.

Default
- Credit bureaus are notified.
- Entire balance becomes due immediately.
- Additional charges, fees, and collection costs are assigned.
- Credit is negatively affected.
- Wages and tax returns are garnished.
- Social Security and disability benefits are withheld.
- Legal fees and court costs are your responsibility.
- You are ineligible for additional student aid.
- Other federal debt collection methods are used.

Remember!

After you leave medical school, even if you do not receive a bill or repayment notice, payments are required and must be made on your federal student loans. It is your responsibility to stay in touch with your loan servicer(s) and make all payments **ON TIME,** even if you do not receive a bill!

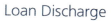

Loan Discharge

Repayment is a serious obligation; however, in certain cases, your federally guaranteed student loans may be discharged and your repayment obligation cancelled or forgiven. Review your promissory note for all terms.

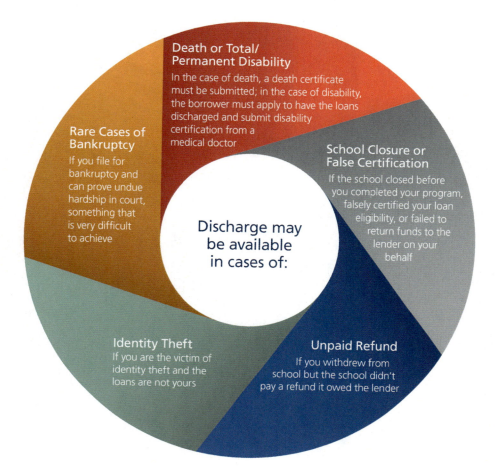

Discharge may be available in cases of:

Death or Total/Permanent Disability
In the case of death, a death certificate must be submitted; in the case of disability, the borrower must apply to have the loans discharged and submit disability certification from a medical doctor

School Closure or False Certification
If the school closed before you completed your program, falsely certified your loan eligibility, or failed to return funds to the lender on your behalf

Unpaid Refund
If you withdrew from school but the school didn't pay a refund it owed the lender

Identity Theft
If you are the victim of identity theft and the loans are not yours

Rare Cases of Bankruptcy
If you file for bankruptcy and can prove undue hardship in court, something that is very difficult to achieve

While you would never want any of these things to happen, if they do, your servicer(s) must be notified so that the appropriate discharge process can begin. For more information, visit StudentAid.gov/manage-loans/forgiveness-cancellation.

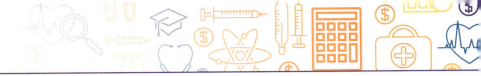

Know the Type of Loans You Borrowed

Important Loan Details

The terms "subsidized" and "unsubsidized" probably sound familiar, but do you know what a subsidy actually is? It's financial assistance that covers accruing interest. The result of a subsidy is that no interest accrues on the loan for the borrower while the subsidy is active. The subsidy only works while you are in school, during qualifying periods of grace and deferment, and during parts of some repayment plans.

As of July 2012, Direct Subsidized Loans are no longer available to graduate or professional students. Therefore, the majority of a medical student's debt will likely be unsubsidized in the form of Direct Unsubsidized Loans. As is the case with any unsubsidized loans, Direct Unsubsidized Loans accrue interest from the date of their disbursement, and payment of that interest will ultimately be the borrower's responsibility.

Subsidized

These loans receive an interest subsidy in which the government or your medical school pays accruing interest on your behalf while you're enrolled in school and during periods of grace and authorized deferment.

- Direct Subsidized
- Perkins*
- Loans for Disadvantaged Students (LDS)*
- Primary Care Loans (PCL)
- Institutional Loans (some)
- Direct Consolidation**

Unsubsidized

These loans accrue interest from the date of disbursement. If the interest is unpaid, it will be added back to the principal balance (original amount borrowed) at specific points via a process called capitalization. You are responsible for this interest.

- Direct Unsubsidized
- Direct PLUS
- Private/Alternative
- Institutional Loans (some)
- Direct Consolidation**

To reduce the cost of interest and capitalization, consider making payments (when possible) toward the interest accruing on your UNSUBSIDIZED loans while you're in school, in grace, in deferment, or in forbearance.

*If consolidated, Perkins and LDS Loans lose their favorable grace and deferment rights and also become unsubsidized balances.

**In a Direct Consolidation Loan, subsidized balances remain subsidized and unsubsidized balances remain unsubsidized — with the exception of Perkins and LDS Loans.

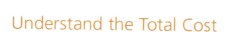

Understand the Total Cost

You have heard the saying that nothing in life is free, and your student loans certainly are no exception. However, understanding exactly how your loans cost you money will help you make smart borrowing and repayment decisions. If your loans are borrowed and paid strategically, you could save yourself time and money.

There are three primary factors that contribute to the cost of your loans:

1. **Interest**
2. **Capitalization**
3. **Length of Repayment**

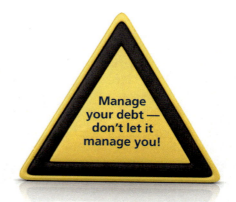

Manage your debt — don't let it manage you!

Interest

The lender charges you to use its money. This charge is known as interest. Understanding the way interest accrues is essential to managing your debt. The most important fact to know about student loan interest is that if the loan is not subsidized, interest accrues on the outstanding principal balance of the loan beginning on the date of disbursement. **You always have the right to pay the accruing interest — even if no payments are required.**

How Interest Accrues on Student Loans

Interest accrues daily on a student loan — from the day it's disbursed until the day the loan balance reaches zero. There is a simple formula to calculate your daily interest accrual:

$$\frac{\text{interest rate (in decimal format)} \times \text{current principal balance}}{\text{number of days in the year}} = \text{daily interest}$$

The day student loans are paid in full, the accrual of interest stops. You only accrue interest on the days you owe a balance, which means that paying off the loans aggressively can save you money in interest.

Furthermore, different loans carry different interest rates. The chart on the next page will help you understand what interest rates have been available in the most recent years for federal student loans.

Student Loan Relief Measures

On April 6, 2022, the U.S. Department of Education extended COVID-19 emergency relief for student loans. This includes 0% interest from March 13, 2020, through Aug. 31, 2022. For more information on student loan relief measures, visit StudentAid.gov/coronavirus.

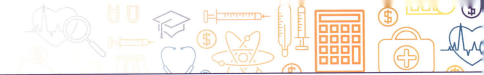

Graduate and Professional Loans*	Interest Rates
Direct Unsubsidized Loans (disbursed between 7/1/22 and 6/30/23)	**6.54%** Fixed
Direct Unsubsidized Loans (disbursed between 7/1/21 and 6/30/22)	**5.28%** Fixed
Direct Unsubsidized Loans (disbursed between 7/1/20 and 6/30/21)	**4.30%** Fixed
Direct Unsubsidized Loans (disbursed between 7/1/19 and 6/30/20)	**6.08%** Fixed
Direct PLUS Loans (disbursed between 7/1/22 and 6/30/23)	**7.54%** Fixed
Direct PLUS Loans (disbursed between 7/1/21 and 6/30/22)	**6.28%** Fixed
Direct PLUS Loans (disbursed between 7/1/20 and 6/30/21)	**5.30%** Fixed
Direct PLUS Loans (disbursed between 7/1/19 and 6/30/20)	**7.08%** Fixed
PCL/LDS	**5.00%** Fixed
Private Loans	**Varies** — Check the Promissory Note
Institutional Loans	**Varies** — Check the Promissory Note
Consolidation Loans	**Fixed rate** based on weighted average interest rate of underlying loans

*For historical interest rate information, visit https://studentaid.gov/understand-aid/types/loans/interest-rates.

Rate Reduction for Automatic Withdrawal

During loan repayment, loans may be eligible for **a 0.25% interest rate reduction**. If you choose to use the automatic debit option for your required payments (after graduation), the loan servicer will automatically deduct your monthly payments from your checking or savings account. Check with your loan servicer to see if this benefit is available.

Debt Management Strategies for Minimizing Interest Costs

Here are some debt management strategies to help you pay your loans off faster:

- **Organize your debt by arranging it from highest to lowest interest rate.** The highest-rate debt should be your first priority.

- **Pay as much as possible toward your highest-rate debt.** Attempt to reduce the required payment on your lower-rate debt — freeing up monies to go to the higher-rate debt.

- **Pay with purpose; it can save you money.** Don't forget to include your credit card and private loan debts in your strategy — they sometimes can be the most expensive debt.

How to Make a Voluntary Payment That Counts

Required and **voluntary payments** can be paid to the loan servicer most easily by accessing your student loan account online at your loan servicer's website. Payments can be made by using the servicer's built-in online payment system. Payments can also be made by sending a check (either a paper one or an electronic check generated from your online bank account). In any case, when sending a voluntary payment, always follow the steps below.

1. Send or submit it separate from any required payment.

2. Include directions telling the servicer which loan the payment should be applied to.

3. Follow up to make sure your payment was applied accurately.

NOTE: During repayment, all fees and interest must be paid before payments can be directed to the principal of the loan. If you fail to provide detailed directions, your servicers can apply the voluntary money to required future payments rather than paying down the current interest.

Capitalization

When the accrued and unpaid interest is added to the original principal of the loan, it is called capitalization. (The principal of a loan is the primary balance you owe, excluding interest and fees.) Capitalization causes your principal balance to increase, and then the capitalized interest begins to accrue interest as well. Capitalization can be costly for a borrower, so it's best if it occurs as infrequently as possible. Some tips to reduce the cost of capitalization are detailed below.

Debt Management Strategies for Minimizing Capitalization

- **Contact the servicers to determine their capitalization policy and verify when your loans are scheduled to capitalize.** This will help you understand what triggers capitalization in your loans, enabling you to avoid unnecessary capitalization. Typically, a medical student's first capitalization occurs at the end of the grace period. After this, additional capitalization of future unpaid interest will depend on which repayment strategy you use to manage the loans.

- **Pay accruing interest prior to capitalization.** This may mean making partial or full interest-only payments while you are in school or residency. Remember, it's always an option to make voluntary payments, even when no payment is required.

- **Submit timely requests.** After you graduate, if you are late filing forms requesting deferment, forbearance, or repayment, capitalization may occur earlier than expected.

Length of Repayment

The length of repayment affects the total cost of the loan. Each repayment plan provides a maximum repayment term, ranging from 10 to 25 years, with a 30-year term possible on consolidation loans. Keep in mind that the ability to prepay a loan, repay on a shorter schedule, or change repayment plans remains available in most situations — just contact the loan servicer. The longer it takes to pay off the loan, the more interest you may pay, and, therefore, the costlier the loan may be. You can choose to make interest-only payments while in school or during residency (if payments have been postponed). To minimize the total cost of student loans, pay the balance off as soon as possible. (Review previous directions for guidance on how to make voluntary payments.)

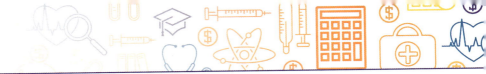

Loan Timeline

During Residency

Let's face it — financially, your years after medical school (residency) will not be your most extravagant or lavish. During this time, not only is it a good idea to continue living within a realistic budget, it is also a good idea to begin actively managing the repayment of your student loans.

Be encouraged. You have many options as you choose the strategy that will best support your financial goals during residency. These options range from postponing payments by using grace, deferment, or forbearance to making reduced (affordable) payments through one of the repayment plans.

Grace

After you leave school, your loans will either enter a grace period or require immediate payment. The grace period is a time when payments aren't required. It occurs automatically. During the grace period, the federal government pays the interest on subsidized loans, not the borrower. Unsubsidized loans continue to accrue interest during the grace period — just as they always have done. The availability and length of a grace period depend on the loan type. The chart on the next page shows some common loans and their grace periods, but notice that Direct PLUS Loans and Consolidation Loans do not offer a grace period — though there are other options available to postpone payments on those loans. Contact your servicers for assistance.

Before Repayment Begins

For many loans, the initial capitalization of accrued interest occurs when you separate from school OR at the end of the grace period. The Loan Repayment Timeline on page 18 depicts when this generally occurs for each loan.

The actual repayment start date for loans differs depending on the:

- Loan type.
- Grace period.
- Loan disbursement date.
- Loan servicer.

It's important to know what's in your loan portfolio and when repayment begins so that you can develop a repayment strategy in a timely manner.

Using Up Your Grace

Many loans enter an automatic grace period after you separate from school; however, you should check with your servicers about your grace period eligibility for each loan because there are numerous ways a grace period can be exhausted (including during any breaks in your education lasting longer than six months). Some loans may offer additional grace periods under certain circumstances, so be sure to check with your servicers.

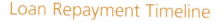

Loan Repayment Timeline

	School	Residency/Graduate Fellowship		Post-Residency
Direct Loan	Enrolled	6-month grace	Deferment,[1] Internship/Residency Forbearance,[2] or Repayment[3]	Repayment[3]
Consolidation Loan	In-School Deferment	Deferment,[1] Internship/Residency Forbearance,[2] or Repayment[3]		Repayment[3]
Direct PLUS Loan[4] Disbursed on or after 7/1/08	In-School Deferment	6-month post-enrollment deferment	Deferment,[1] Internship/Residency Forbearance,[2] or Repayment[3]	Repayment[3]
Perkins Loan	Enrolled	9-month grace	Deferment,[1] Forbearance,[5] or Repayment.[3] Possible 6-month post-deferment grace.	Repayment[3]
Primary Care Loan	Enrolled	12-month grace	Residency Deferment (up to 4 years in an eligible primary care residency program) Must reapply each year	Repayment[3]
Loans for Disadvantaged Students (LDS)	Enrolled	12-month grace	Deferment available throughout residency Must reapply each year	Repayment[3]
Institutional Loan	Enrolled	Possible Grace, Deferment, or Forbearance. Consult your financial aid office; check promissory note.		Repayment[3]
Private Loan	Enrolled	Possible Grace, Deferment, or Forbearance Varies by lender; check promissory note		Repayment[3]

1. The FSA website provides a chart of possible deferments and forbearances at StudentAid.gov/manage-loans/lower-payments/get-temporary-relief.
2. Internship/Residency Forbearance: Available on Direct Subsidized and Unsubsidized Loans, Direct PLUS Loans, and Direct Consolidation Loans. This forbearance allows you to postpone or reduce the amount of your monthly payment for a limited and specific period of time if you have been accepted into an internship/residency program.
3. Repayment: Consult with your servicer about repayment plans and postponement options that may be available.
4. Direct PLUS Loans disbursed before July 1, 2008, are not eligible for post-enrollment deferment. Direct PLUS Loans disbursed on or after July 1, 2008, receive an automatic six-month post-enrollment deferment. Contact the servicer for payment or postponement options.
5. Perkins Loans only: Upon receipt of written request and documentation, an institution must grant a temporary postponement of payments for up to one year at a time, not to exceed a total of three years.

This timeline is intended to provide general information and is subject to change based on federal regulations. Always consult your servicer for detailed information about grace, deferment, forbearance, and repayment options.

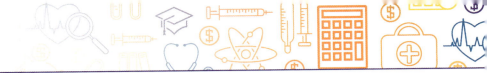

Postponing Payments

While you are enrolled in school at least half-time, payments are not required on any of your federal student loans. Payments are postponed automatically while you are a student through either an in-school status or an in-school deferment that is applied to your loans. After graduating or separating from medical school, there are several other ways to continue to postpone payments. Keep in mind that if at any time you cannot make a required payment, you should contact your servicers immediately and ask them to help you identify postponement options.

Deferment

Deferment is a period of time when a borrower who meets certain criteria can delay making payments. During a deferment, the government pays the interest that accrues on subsidized loans. For unsubsidized loans, the borrower remains responsible for interest accruing during a deferment.

Deferment does not occur automatically; you must apply AND qualify to receive a deferment. As a medical school graduate, it can be difficult to qualify for most types of deferment, but it is possible in some circumstances. The following deferments exist:

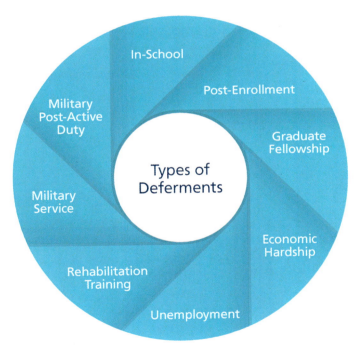

As a resident, the likelihood of qualifying for a deferment is limited, but on that same note, since the majority of current medical school graduates have few to no subsidized loans, the value of a deferment (in the form of subsidies) is minimal, or none at all. If you think you may qualify for a deferment, contact your servicer to discuss eligibility and application procedures. If you have more than one servicer, you will need to contact each one.

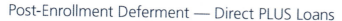

Post-Enrollment Deferment — Direct PLUS Loans

Officially, Direct PLUS Loans enter repayment immediately after they are fully disbursed. However, servicers will automatically apply an in-school deferment on your Direct PLUS Loans to postpone payments while you are enrolled in school.

After you leave school, although no grace period is available, a six-month post-enrollment deferment will be applied automatically to the loan. This deferment mimics a grace period in that it postpones payments for six months, and since Direct PLUS Loans are unsubsidized, interest will accrue during this time. If you prefer to start repayment immediately — to avoid the additional accrual of interest — contact your servicers to decline this deferment.

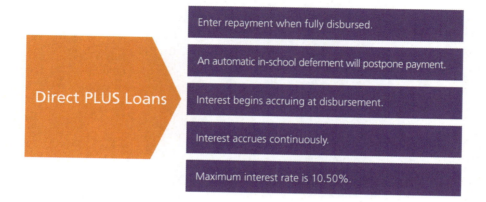

Direct PLUS Loans

- Enter repayment when fully disbursed.
- An automatic in-school deferment will postpone payment.
- Interest begins accruing at disbursement.
- Interest accrues continuously.
- Maximum interest rate is 10.50%.

Forbearance

This status is where most medical school graduates will find the solution to their postponement requests. Forbearance is the period of time when a borrower may either:

- Make reduced payments.
- Postpone required payments.

During forbearance, interest accrues on ALL loans, including subsidized loans — potentially making it a costly option. Though, you can voluntarily pay accruing interest during a forbearance, but interest left unpaid will capitalize. This capitalization typically occurs at the end of the forbearance period; however, according to regulation, capitalization is allowed to occur as often as each quarter, so check with your servicers for their capitalization policies.

All forbearance periods must be formally requested from the loan servicer, who, in most cases, will determine the type and length of the forbearance. For medical interns and residents, several forbearance types are available, but the type most often used is a mandatory forbearance (described next).

Despite forbearance periods allowing the postponement of required payments, a borrower always has the right, and option, to send voluntary payments to the loan servicer — even during a forbearance. Actions like this (voluntary payments) may help to minimize the total repayment cost. To learn about your forbearance options, contact your servicers.

Mandatory Forbearance for Medical Interns and Residents

Medical interns and residents are eligible for a mandatory forbearance on their federal student loans. Although you must first request and provide documentation of your eligibility as a medical intern or resident, once you have done this, the servicer is required to grant the forbearance on your federal loans. This mandatory forbearance is approved in annual increments; therefore, reapplication is necessary each year to keep the forbearance active for the duration of residency.

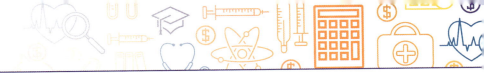

If the application for the next increment of forbearance is done in a timely manner, 30 days before the current increment expires, then capitalization will be delayed until the last increment of forbearance expires. In this manner, you could not only postpone payments throughout residency, you could also postpone the capitalization of the unpaid interest.

Forbearance provisions may differ on some loans, such as the federal Perkins Loan that requires you to pay at least some interest while in forbearance. Be sure to find out from your servicers what the provisions are on your loans. During forbearance, interest accrues on the entire loan balance, but you can always make voluntary payments without losing the forbearance status.

The Cost to Postpone*

For a 2022 graduate with $200,000 in Direct Loans, the capitalization of interest accrued during school and grace will result in a principal balance of $213,600. During residency, an estimated $1,100 in interest will accrue on this balance each month.

Reflects 0% interest from March 13, 2020, to Jan. 31, 2022.

MEDICAL STUDENT EDUCATION ✓ DEBT AND COSTS

2021 GRADUATES WITH MEDICAL EDUCATION DEBT

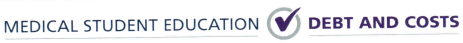

PUBLIC SCHOOLS
74%
Median debt:
$195,000

PRIVATE SCHOOLS
70%
Median debt:
$220,000

ALL
73%
Median debt:
$200,000

MEDIAN 4-YEAR COST OF ATTENDANCE, CLASS OF 2022

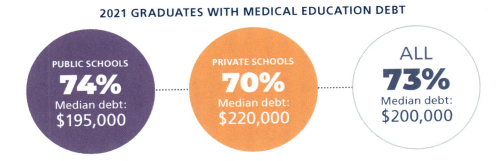

PUBLIC $263,488

PRIVATE $357,868

ALL 2021 GRADUATES

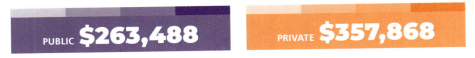

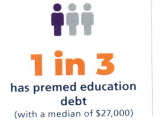

1 in 3
has premed education debt
(with a median of $27,000)

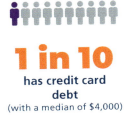

1 in 10
has credit card debt
(with a median of $4,000)

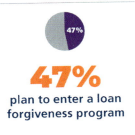

47%

47%
plan to enter a loan forgiveness program

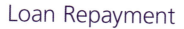

Loan Repayment

When to Start Paying and How Much

For students enrolled at least half-time, payments are not required on federal student loans during medical school. If you are disciplined with your finances during medical school and residency, you will find that the task of repaying your loans may be easier. By making smart financial decisions early and consistently, you can significantly reduce the cost of your debt and the length of time it takes to repay your loans.

Debt Management Fact
The faster you reduce the principal of your loans, the less your debt will cost you.

Direct Unsubsidized Loans, Perkins Loans, and other loans with a grace period will enter repayment at the end of the grace period. In the case of Direct PLUS Loans, payment is required after the post-enrollment deferment ends. For loans without a grace period, you will be required to begin repayment when you graduate, withdraw, or drop below half-time status. See the Loan Repayment Timeline on page 18 for more details.

Approximately one to two months before your first payment is due, you will receive a notice about the exact due date. Around that same time, if not earlier, you'll also be asked to select a repayment plan. The plan you opt for will determine the amount of your required monthly payment and, consequently, the amount of interest you will pay over the life of the loan. Understanding the repayment plans will enable you to choose the best plan for your financial situation.

Rights During Repayment

Take comfort in knowing that if your financial situation changes, you have the ability and the right to request any of the following:

- Deferment or forbearance to postpone payments.
- Changes in the repayment plan (which can change the required monthly payment amount).
- Shortening of the repayment schedule.
- Prepayment of loans without penalty.

Contact your servicers as your circumstance requires.

Get a Jump on Your Loan Payments

It may be a relief to know that you don't have to make payments during school or residency if you don't want to, but you may want to consider making some type of payment — especially toward your most expensive (that is, highest interest rate) debt.

Making interest payments while in residency can be a very smart thing to do because each dollar you pay now helps reduce the overall cost of your debt. The quicker you pay off your debt, the less it may cost you.

NOTE: *You can make payments toward federal student loans at any time, without penalty. Your grace, deferment, or forbearance status will remain uninterrupted even after a voluntary payment is made.*

aamc.org/FIRST

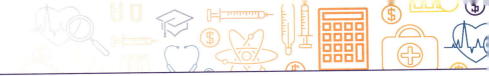

Repayment Plans: Overview

You have various repayment plans to choose from for repaying your federal student loans. The purpose of the different repayment plans is to provide flexibility in your finances. **In most cases, you can change the selected plan when your financial situation changes.**

Repayment plans can be broken down into two groups: the traditional plans and the income-driven plans. Whether your debt is large or small, the repayment plan you select will affect the total cost of the loans. A hasty decision could turn out to be a costly choice, so when the time comes, consider your financial goals and select your repayment plan wisely.

For New Borrowers on or after July 1, 2014:

If you choose the new borrower IBR plan as your repayment plan, your monthly payment amount will be the same as the PAYE monthly payment amount. However, the interest capitalization policy mirrors the original IBR (meaning there is no limit to the amount that capitalizes). Review the information about IBR and PAYE on pages 26-29.

Traditional Plans

Standard Repayment	$2,400/mo
Extended Repayment	$1,400/mo
Graduated Repayment	$1,000/mo (for 2 years)

Income-Driven Plans

Income-Contingent Repayment (ICR)	$780/mo
Income-Based Repayment (IBR)*	$500/mo
Pay As You Earn (PAYE)	$330/mo
Revised Pay As You Earn (REPAYE)	$330/mo

Based on an original balance of $200,000, entering repayment after four years of medical school and six months of grace. ICR, IBR, PAYE, and REPAYE are based on a stipend of $59,300. *(Values are rounded to the nearest $10 and reflect the effects of student loan relief measures, March 13, 2020-Jan. 31, 2022, where appropriate.)*

*Borrowers who possessed student loans before July 1, 2014, are eligible for only the original IBR plan modeled in this chart. If you had no outstanding student loans when you received your first Direct Loan on or after July 1, 2014, then you are considered a "new borrower" and are eligible for the new IBR plan, which mirrors the PAYE payment amounts.

aamc.org/FIRST

Traditional Repayment Plans

Traditional repayment plans are based on formulas that look only at the amount of debt owed. These plans can save you money during repayment because they are designed to fully repay the loans within a specific period of time. Keep in mind that the longer the term, the higher the cost of repayment, because more interest is allowed to accrue. When a borrower makes higher monthly payments, less interest accrues and the total cost of the loan can be less. Traditional repayment plans are Standard, Extended, and Graduated, all of which are detailed in the following pages.

Standard Repayment

When you choose this plan, your monthly payment amount will generally be the same throughout the term of the loan, which is typically 10 years. Compared with the other options, the Standard plan requires higher monthly payments but results in lower interest costs. Standard Repayment allows borrowers to pay education debt in an aggressive and cost-efficient manner.

If you fail to notify your servicers of a repayment plan choice, you will automatically be signed up for the Standard Repayment plan.

 Best option for borrowers whose primary goal is minimizing the total interest cost of their student loan debt.

Extended Repayment

The Extended Repayment plan allows you to stretch your current repayment term up to 25 years, which lowers the required monthly payment. To qualify for Extended Repayment, you must have an outstanding balance of principal and interest totaling more than $30,000.

Before opting to extend your repayment term, consider the degree to which this option will increase the total interest cost of your debt.

 Best option for borrowers seeking to lower their required monthly payment (without consolidating or exhibiting a Partial Financial Hardship — refer to page 26).

Graduated Repayment

The Graduated Repayment plan allows you to begin making smaller monthly payments during the first two years of repayment, then significantly higher monthly payments for the remaining eight years of a 10-year repayment term. Often, the initial payment amount in this plan is equal to the amount of interest that accrues monthly, making it potentially an interest-only payment plan during those first few years.

Even though Graduated Repayment offers monthly payments that start lower than the Standard Repayment amount, this plan can lead to higher interest costs because the principal of the loan is not paid off as quickly. Additionally, in the third year of this plan, the payment may increase dramatically. For these reasons, this is not a plan that medical residents tend to select.

Best option for borrowers seeking temporary relief from high loan payments but expecting an increase in their income shortly after repayment begins.

Income-Driven Repayment Plans

Income-driven repayment plans offer affordable payments on federal student loans because they are based on income and family size. However, the affordability of these payments can lead to higher costs — sometimes significantly higher — because interest may be allowed to accrue for longer. In certain cases, these plans will result in forgiveness of the balance at the end of the term, currently a taxable forgiveness. In addition to forgiveness based on the term of the plans, all income-driven plans also qualify for Public Service Loan Forgiveness (PSLF), which is currently not taxable. Income-driven plans include Income-Contingent Repayment (ICR), two versions of Income-Based Repayment (IBR), Pay As You Earn (PAYE), and Revised Pay As You Earn (REPAYE).

Income-Contingent Repayment (ICR)*

The Income-Contingent Repayment (ICR) plan is an income-driven plan that is based on 20% of your discretionary income. When income is low, such as during residency, the ICR plan will require payments that are lower than the payments in traditional repayment plans. Compared with the other income-driven plans, ICR payment amounts will be greater. Additionally, while in ICR, there is no maximum for the payment amount. Therefore, as your salary increases, your ICR payment will also increase. Considering the earning potential of a physician, the ICR plan could lead to one of the highest monthly payment amounts, but this in turn could also result in the ICR plan being one of the lowest total repayment cost options.

As with the other income-driven plans, annual income documentation is needed to determine the monthly payment. This payment will be adjusted annually based on changes to your household income. Since the ICR plan has a higher required payment than the other income-driven plans, the IBR plans, PAYE, or REPAYE may offer additional financial flexibility with lower payments.

The maximum repayment term for ICR is 25 years. After that, any unpaid balance is forgiven (but will be taxable). Although ICR qualifies for PSLF, it may be more beneficial to use a repayment plan that has a lower monthly payment, allowing for more monies to be forgiven via the PSLF program.

★ **Best option for borrowers who want a payment that is affordable when income is low but would prefer to minimize the total interest cost of student loan debt as soon as their income increases.**

*ICR is available only for loans originally disbursed by Direct Loans. Federal Family Education Loan (FFEL) Program loans have a similar plan, referred to as Income-Sensitive Repayment. Speak to your FFEL servicers for more details.

Income-Based Repayment (IBR)*

The Income-Based Repayment (IBR) plan is available for all federal loan borrowers who exhibit a Partial Financial Hardship (PFH). The loan servicers will determine if a PFH exists, but most medical residents exhibit this hardship.

In the IBR plan, the monthly payment is equal to and capped at 15% of discretionary income. The monthly IBR payment is adjusted annually according to changes in household income and family size. This plan offers a partial interest subsidy that is only available for the first three years of the plan. For subsidized loan borrowers during this time, the federal government will pay the amount of interest that accrues on the subsidized loans that exceeds the IBR payment amount. Capitalization of all the unpaid interest will not occur until after the PFH ceases to exist or until the borrower elects to leave IBR. Since many residents will show a PFH throughout residency, capitalization could be postponed until residency is over, if not longer. There is no limit to how much interest can capitalize under IBR.

What Is a Partial Financial Hardship (PFH)?

A PFH exists when the 10-year standard monthly payment on what you owe when you first enter repayment is more than 15% (if entering IBR) or 10% (if entering PAYE) of your discretionary income. **Discretionary income** is the difference between your income and 150% of the poverty guideline (based on your family size and state of residence).

The IBR payment amount adjusts annually based on household income and family size — **so be sure to provide your servicers with updated information each year in a timely manner.** The IBR plan has a maximum payment amount, meaning that no matter how much your income increases in future years, you cannot be "kicked out" of the plan. Required payments in the IBR plans will never exceed what the 10-year Standard Repayment amount would have been (based on the debt amount that was initially brought into the plan). This maximum payment will be required when you no longer show a PFH.

If you pay under IBR for 25 years, any remaining balance that exists after this time will be forgiven (and taxed), though many physicians are likely to have fully repaid their loans before reaching this point. This plan also qualifies as an eligible plan for Public Service Loan Forgiveness (PSLF). With PSLF, the forgiven amount is not taxable.

★ **Best option for borrowers with lower salaries experiencing a financial hardship and/or for those seeking some type of loan forgiveness.**

*Borrowers who have balances on federal student loans received before July 1, 2014, are eligible for only the original IBR plan, as discussed above. If a borrower had no outstanding student loan balance before July 1, 2014, then they are considered a "new borrower" and are eligible for the new IBR plan, which mirrors the PAYE payment amounts. However, the interest capitalization policy of the new IBR plan mimics that of the original IBR plan (meaning there is no limit to the amount that can capitalize).

The Partial Financial Hardship (PFH) test for entering IBR or PAYE:

IS YOUR STANDARD MONTHLY PAYMENT . . .
(the 10-year monthly payment amount determined when you enter the plan)

greater than > **your monthly payment in IBR or PAYE** ?
(whichever plan you are applying for)

If "yes," you have a PFH.

FOR EXAMPLE . . .
For a medical student who borrowed $200,000 of federal student loans and a PGY-1 stipend of $59,700* . . .

the Standard monthly payment would be **$2,360** > the IBR monthly payment would be **$500**

or

the PAYE monthly payment would be **$330**

. . . you will see that the borrower has a PFH and meets the requirement to qualify for IBR or PAYE since the borrower's Standard monthly payment would be greater than payment under IBR or PAYE.

*Based on the AAMC estimate for the 2022 first post-MD-year median stipend.

Example of a PGY-1 Resident		
	In IBR	In PAYE
Monthly Adjusted Gross Income[1]	$4,980	$4,980
(minus) 150% of Poverty Line[2]	− $1,640	− $1,640
Discretionary Income[3]	= $3,340	= $3,340
(multiplied by)[4]	× 15%	× 10%
Monthly Payment[5]	$500	$330

1. Based on AAMC estimate for the 2022 first post-MD-year median stipend.
2. Based on the 2022 federal poverty guideline for a family size of one in the 48 contiguous states.
3. Discretionary income is the difference between your income and 150% of the poverty guideline (based on your family size and state of residence).
4. Based on 2015 federal regulations.
5. Rounded to the nearest $10.

NOTE: If you're a new borrower on or after July 1, 2014, the "new" IBR payment plan amount will be equal to the PAYE amount, but the capitalization policy will mirror the original IBR (that is, there will be no limit to how much interest can capitalize). This means that the PAYE plan may lead to a lower total repayment cost.

IBR for New Borrowers (as of July 1, 2014)

Another version of the IBR plan is now available for new federal loan borrowers who began borrowing on or after July 1, 2014. Under this more recent version of IBR, you must still show a Partial Financial Hardship (PFH) to enter the plan. Just like the original IBR plan, the new IBR plan adjusts payments annually, provides a partial interest subsidy for the first three years, and capitalizes unpaid interest — with no limit to the amount that capitalizes. This repayment plan also qualifies for Public Service Loan Forgiveness (PSLF).

The primary difference between the original and the new IBR plans is that the new IBR plan will have payments capped at 10% of discretionary income, rather than 15% — likely making the new-borrower IBR plan more affordable than the original IBR plan.

Additionally, if you pay under the new IBR plan for 20 years (rather than 25 years, as the original IBR requires), any remaining balance will be forgiven (but is taxable). Obtaining a "term" forgiveness with the new IBR plan is more likely since the term is shorter.

Although similar to PAYE, the new IBR plan will likely cost more in interest than the PAYE plan because interest accrual is limited inside PAYE, while the new IBR plan has no limit on accrued interest. The limited interest accrual of the PAYE plan makes it preferable to the new IBR plan.

Pay As You Earn (PAYE)*

Pay As You Earn (PAYE) is similar to the IBR plans in that it is only available for those experiencing a Partial Financial Hardship (PFH) — refer to page 26 for more details on PFH. Since many medical residents exhibit a PFH throughout residency, it can be easy for a resident to enter and remain in the PAYE plan throughout residency and beyond. For subsidized loan borrowers, an interest subsidy is available for the first three years in this plan and covers the interest accruing on the subsidized loans that is greater than the PAYE payment amount.

Unlike the original IBR plan that calculates payments as 15% of discretionary income, the PAYE plan bases monthly payments on 10% of discretionary income — making the PAYE payments lower than the original IBR plan payments. Furthermore, the amount of unpaid interest that can capitalize under the PAYE plan is equal to 10% of the loan balance that entered into this plan. Once the maximum amount has capitalized, interest will continue to accrue, but it will not be capitalized.

PAYE Tips

To qualify for PAYE, you must:

1. Be a new borrower on or after Oct. 1, 2007 (meaning you owed no federal loans as of this date)

AND

2. Have received a Direct Loan disbursement on or after Oct. 1, 2011.

Not sure if you owed loans as of Oct. 1, 2007?

Log in to your FSA account at StudentAid.gov to see the date you received each loan.

For a qualified medical resident, there are several reasons to choose PAYE:

1. Partial interest subsidy (free money available only for those with subsidized loans).

2. Limit to the amount capitalized after entering the plan and a potential postponement of capitalization.

3. Capped maximum payment amount.

4. Several possible forgiveness programs.

5. Potentially the lowest required payment amount during residency.

The PAYE payment amount adjusts annually based on household income and family size; however, no matter how much income increases, the PAYE payment is capped at a predetermined amount. This maximum amount cannot exceed what the 10-year Standard Repayment amount would have been (based on the debt amount when the borrower entered the PAYE plan). The maximum payment is required when the PFH ceases to exist.

The repayment term for PAYE is up to 20 years. After that, any unpaid balance is forgiven (and is taxable). This plan also qualifies as an eligible payment plan for Public Service Loan Forgiveness (PSLF).

★ **Best option for qualified borrowers with a lower income who are experiencing a financial hardship and/or seeking some type of loan forgiveness.**

*Only Direct Loans are eligible.

Revised Pay As You Earn (REPAYE)*

In 2015, a version of the PAYE plan called Revised Pay As You Earn (REPAYE) was made available for federal student loan borrowers. The purpose of REPAYE is to provide more student loan borrowers access to the affordable terms of the income-driven plans. REPAYE accomplishes this by providing lenient terms:

- **There are no** income requirements.
- A Partial Financial Hardship (PFH) is not needed to enter the plan.
- The loan disbursement dates do not affect the borrower's eligibility.

REPAYE allows borrowers who do not qualify for PAYE or IBR to make affordable monthly payments (equal to 10% of their discretionary income). REPAYE payments adjust annually based on the most recent income — adjusted gross income (AGI) or modified adjusted gross income (MAGI) — as reported on one's taxes filed for the previous year.

For subsidized loans, in REPAYE, borrowers are not responsible for the remaining accrued interest after the regular monthly payment has been applied. This condition exists during the first three consecutive years of repayment and is a feature applicable only to subsidized loans in REPAYE and, thus, offers no benefit to borrowers who have no subsidized loans in their debt portfolio. After the first three years of repayment is over, borrowers are then only responsible for 50% of the accrued but unpaid interest on the subsidized loans after the regular monthly payment has been applied. For unsubsidized loans, the policy is slightly different: For the entire REPAYE payment period, borrowers are only responsible for 50% of the accrued interest that's not covered by their regular monthly payment amount — the other half is subsidized by the U.S. Department of Education.

REPAYE payments qualify for Public Service Loan Forgiveness (PSLF), and loan forgiveness is available for graduate-level students after 25 years of payments (rather than 20 years with PAYE). Currently, the amount forgiven is taxable.

★ **Best option for borrowers who are seeking lower required monthly payments and/or some type of loan forgiveness.**

*Only Direct Loans are eligible.

Married Borrowers and Income-Driven Repayment Plans

Marriage can affect student loan repayment for medical graduates. Some plans, including the traditional repayment plans, are unaffected by a borrower's marital status. Other plans, like the income-driven repayment plans, are severely altered. To calculate the impact that marriage may have on student loan repayment for you (and your spouse), use the MedLoans Organizer and Calculator (MLOC) at aamc.org/medloans.

Below is an overview of how a borrower's change in marital status, from single to married, may affect certain income-driven repayments plans.

Impact of a Spouse's Income

The effect of a spouse's income on repayment differs by plan. Several of the income-driven plans only factor in your spouse's income in certain situations, while other income-driven repayment plans always consider both your income and your spouse's income.

Revised Pay As You Earn (REPAYE) — In REPAYE, although eligibility to enter REPAYE is unaffected by a spouse's earnings, both your income and your spouse's income are used to determine your monthly loan payment. This is the case whether you and your spouse file your federal income taxes jointly or separately.

Pay As You Earn (PAYE), Income-Based Repayment (IBR), and Income-Contingent Repayment (ICR) — In these income-driven plans, how the servicer looks at your spouse's income will depend on your tax filing status. If you file separately, your servicer will only use your income (the borrower) to determine both your eligibility for the plan and the amount of your monthly payment. If you file jointly, both your income and your spouse's incomes will be factored into your eligibility and payment amount for these repayment plans.

Check with a tax advisor to determine whether you and your spouse should file jointly or separately because this decision can affect more than just your student loan payments.

Impact of a Spouse's Debt

A spouse's federal student loan debt is treated in the same manner as their income: Certain plans add it into the household's debt, while others may ignore it.

REPAYE — Loan servicers will always determine your monthly payment (and your spouse's) based on joint income and debt; however, the amount that each spouse owes their servicer is proportionate to how much of the total debt is theirs. Here is an example provided by the Department of Education: If the calculated REPAYE payment amount for you and your spouse (based on your joint income) is $200, and you owe 60% of your combined loan debt and your spouse owes 40%, your individual REPAYE payment would be $120, and your spouse's individual REPAYE payment would be $80. So, when a married couple is told how much the household owes, it does not mean that each spouse owes that amount but rather that each spouse owes a proportionate amount of the payment to their servicer(s).

PAYE or IBR — In PAYE or IBR, your spouse's federal student loan debt and income are ignored if you and your spouse file your taxes separately. If you file jointly, your spouse's income and debt are factored into determining the repayment plan payment amount.

Repayment Plans Compared: Which One Works for You?

	Traditional Plans			Income-Contingent Repayment (ICR)
	Standard	**Extended**	**Graduated**	
Available in Which Loan Program?	Direct and FFEL	Direct and FFEL	Direct and FFEL	Direct only
What Are the Advantages of This Plan?	May provide the lowest total repayment cost (due to less interest accruing)	Reduced monthly payment, without consolidating	Can offer temporary relief to borrowers expecting an income increase in the near future	Payments may initially be lower than traditional plan payments but will increase as income increases. Capitalized interest cannot exceed 10% of the loan amount that enters the plan. After this, interest accrues but does not capitalize.
How Is the Monthly Payment Determined?	Payments calculated equally over the repayment term; payment based on total amount owed	Equal monthly payments stretched over a longer term; payment based on total amount owed	Payments begin lower (interest only in the first 2 years of a 10-year term) and then increase.	Payments are based on the lesser of 20% of your monthly discretionary income or your monthly payment on a 12-year plan times a percentage factor based on your income.
What Is the Repayment Term?	10 years (up to 30 years if consolidated)	25 years	10 years (up to 30 years if consolidated)	Up to 25 years (after which any remaining balance is forgiven but will be taxable)
What Are the Eligibility Requirements?	Plan available upon request	Must owe more than $30,000 in Direct Loans or FFEL	Available upon request	No initial income eligibility. Payments are based on income and family size.
Does It Qualify for PSLF?	Yes	No	No	Yes
What Else Should You Know About This Plan?	This is the default plan if no other plan is selected. A consolidation loan must be repaid on a 10-year Standard plan (or an income-driven plan) to qualify for PSLF.	This plan will generally cost more than the other traditional plans due to the longer repayment term and the resulting increase in interest costs.	The minimum payment is interest only, which can result in higher interest costs compared with the Standard plan.	Income and family size must be verified annually; no cap on the maximum payment amount.

aamc.org/FIRST

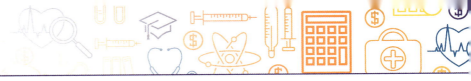

Income-Driven Plans			
Income-Based Repayment (IBR) (for those who borrowed before July 1, 2014)	**Income-Based Repayment (IBR) (for new borrowers as of July 1, 2014)**	**Pay As You Earn (PAYE)**	**Revised Pay As You Earn (REPAYE)**
Direct and FFEL	Direct only	Direct only	Direct only
Provides affordable payments based on family size and adjusted gross income (AGI) for the household, but there is no limit to interest capitalization	Payments mirror the PAYE payments, but there is no limit to interest capitalization.	May allow for the lowest possible monthly payment. Capitalization cannot exceed 10% of the loan amount that enters the plan. After reaching this limit, interest will accrue but does not capitalize.	May allow for the lowest possible monthly payment. When the monthly payment doesn't cover the interest, you are responsible for only 50% of the accrued and unpaid interest.
Payments are calculated at 15% of your monthly discretionary income and are based on your family size and AGI for the household. The amount is capped at the 10-year Standard payment amount (determined when you enter IBR).	Payments are calculated at 10% of your monthly discretionary income and are based on your family size and AGI for the household. The amount is capped at the 10-year Standard payment amount (determined when you enter IBR).	Payments are calculated at 10% of your monthly discretionary income and are based on your family size and AGI for the household. The amount is capped at the 10-year Standard payment amount (determined when you enter PAYE).	Payments are calculated at 10% of your monthly discretionary income and are based on your family size and AGI for the household. There is no cap on the maximum payment amount.
Up to 25 years (after which any remaining balance is forgiven but will be taxable)	Up to 20 years (after which any remaining balance is forgiven but will be taxable)	Up to 20 years (after which any remaining balance is forgiven but will be taxable)	Up to 25 years for a graduate-level student borrower (after which any remaining balance is forgiven but will be taxable)
Must have a Partial Financial Hardship (PFH) to qualify	Must be a new borrower on or after July 1, 2014, and also have a PFH to qualify	Must have a PFH, be a new borrower on or after Oct. 1, 2007, and have a Direct Loan disbursement on or after Oct. 1, 2011. Available only for Direct Loans.	Available only for Direct Loans. There are no additional eligibility requirements.
Yes	Yes	Yes	Yes
Income and family size must be verified annually; payments can be as low as $0/month. If filing taxes jointly, spouse's income will be considered in eligibility and payment amounts.	Income and family size must be verified annually; payments can be as low as $0/month. If filing taxes jointly, spouse's income will be considered in eligibility and payment amounts.	Income and family size must be verified annually; payments can be as low as $0/month. If filing taxes jointly, spouse's income will be considered in eligibility and payment amounts.	No cap on the maximum payment or on the amount of interest that can capitalize. Income and family size must be verified annually; payments can be as low as $0/month. Spouse's income is always factored into determining the monthly payment.

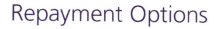

Repayment Options

To Pay or Not to Pay

After medical school, residents choose between two options to manage their federal education loans: making payments or postponing payments. To quickly understand the financial impact of each option, compare the results of the case studies detailed in the following pages.

Making Payments During Residency

If you choose to pay during residency, the most feasible plan will likely be either the PAYE or the REPAYE plan. These plans offer similar benefits along with affordable monthly payments, as seen in the following case studies. The case studies are based on repaying four different debt levels during a four year-residency. Reviewing the one that most closely resembles your debt level can help clarify your situation.

Keep in mind, you can switch between repayment plans and adjust your repayment strategy at any time; however, it is important to understand that capitalization will occur for any unpaid accrued interest (when you change plans). You can also make extra payments no matter what plan you choose. To make extra (voluntary) payments, follow the instructions on page 16.

Would you like to view personalized repayment scenarios? Use the MedLoans® Organizer and Calculator (MLOC) at aamc.org/medloans to see numbers and repayment results based on your loan portfolio, family size, time in training, and future income amounts. Login details for the MLOC are available on page 6. NOTE: At this time, the MLOC allows you to calculate the impact of different repayment plans and forgiveness options, but not to calculate the impact for scenarios where you make additional payments. To see the positive impact extra payments can have on your total cost and time to repay, review the case studies on pages 35-38.

Postponing Payments During Residency

Residents who choose to postpone payments will likely do so by requesting a Mandatory Medical Residency Forbearance from their loan servicer. The following case studies show the impact of postponing payments and then choosing a variety of post-residency repayment options. Federal student loan borrowers always have the right to prepay their loans without penalty. Even when no payments are required, you can still send voluntary payments to your loan servicers. Refer to page 16 for more details on how to make a voluntary payment.

Keep in mind, you have the right to switch into and out of a Mandatory Medical Residency Forbearance or to change repayment plans. To do so, contact your loan servicer. **Be advised that when the status of your loans change (like switching repayment plans or going into or out of a forbearance), the capitalization of unpaid interest will occur. It is important to determine whether the desired change outweighs the impact of unnecessary capitalization.**

The lower the monthly payment, the higher the total interest cost.

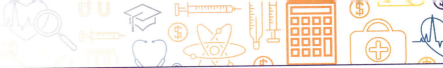

Debt-Level Case Studies During Residency

Case Study No. 1: $150,000 Borrowed and $250,000 Post-Residency Salary

PAYE Payments During a Four-Year Residency

Monthly Payment During Residency	Repayment Plan: **PAYE**	Repayment Years After Residency	Estimated Monthly Payment After Residency	Interest Cost	Total Repayment
$330 to $410	During and after residency	11.6	$1,800	$112,000	$262,000
$330 to $410	During residency, then Standard	6	$3,200	$99,000	$249,000
$330 to $410	During and after residency + additional $500/mo after residency	8.3	$2,300	$93,000	$243,000
$330 to $410	During and after residency + additional $1,000/mo after residency	6.5	$2,800	$82,000	$232,000

REPAYE Payments During a Four-Year Residency

Monthly Payment During Residency	Repayment Plan: **REPAYE**	Repayment Years After Residency	Estimated Monthly Payment After Residency	Interest Cost	Total Repayment
$330 to $410	During and after residency	7.8	$2,100 to $2,500	$79,000	$229,000
$330 to $410	During residency, then Standard	6	$2,800	$69,000	$219,000
$330 to $410	During and after residency + additional $500/mo after residency*	6.2	$2,600 to $2,900	$70,000	$220,000
$330 to $410	During and after residency + additional $1,000/mo after residency*	5.2	$3,100 to $3,400	$64,000	$214,000

Forbearance During a Four-Year Residency

Monthly Payment During Residency	Repayment Plan	Repayment Years After Residency	Estimated Monthly Payment After Residency	Interest Cost	Total Repayment
$0	Standard + pay extra each month to pay off in five years after residency	5	$3,800	$77,000	$227,000
$0	Standard	10	$2,200	$108,000	$258,000
$0	Extended	25	$1,200	$217,000	$367,000
$0	PAYE	10.1	$2,100 to $2,200	$109,000	$259,000
$0	REPAYE	9.2	$2,100 to $2,600	$105,000	$255,000

*When sending additional payments, the maximum monthly payment reached may be lower than expected (when simply adding the additional payment to the first row's maximum) because the loans will be paid off before reaching that maximum level.

Note: Values for repayment years and dollar amounts were rounded and are based on a 0% interest from March 13, 2020, through Jan. 31, 2022. Payments during residency are based on an average resident's stipend and a family size of one.

Use the MedLoans Organizer and Calculator to see the full impact of these repayment options on your loan portfolio.

Case Study No. 2: $200,000 Borrowed and $250,000 Post-Residency Salary

PAYE Payments During a Four-Year Residency

Monthly Payment During Residency	Repayment Plan: **PAYE**	Repayment Years After Residency	Estimated Monthly Payment After Residency	Interest Cost	Total Repayment
$330 to $410	During and after residency	12.6	$2,100 to $2,400	$164,000	$364,000
$330 to $410	During residency then Standard	6	$4,100	$110,000	$310,000
$330 to $410	During and after residency + additional $500/mo after residency	9.7	$2,600 to $2,900	$139,000	$339,000
$330 to $410	During and after residency + additional $1,000/mo after residency	7.8	$3,100 to $3,400	$124,000	$324,000

REPAYE Payments During a Four-Year Residency

Monthly Payment During Residency	Repayment Plan: **REPAYE**	Repayment Years After Residency	Estimated Monthly Payment After Residency	Interest Cost	Total Repayment
$330 to $410	During and after residency	11.2	$2,100 to $2,700	$134,000	$334,000
$330 to $410	During residency then Standard	6	$3,800	$92,000	$292,000
$330 to $410	During and after residency + additional $500/mo after residency*	8.8	$2,600 to $3,000	$114,000	$314,000
$330 to $410	During and after residency + additional $1,000/mo after residency*	7.3	$3,100 to $3,500	$101,000	$301,000

Forbearance During a Four-Year Residency

Monthly Payment During Residency	Repayment Plan	Repayment Years After Residency	Estimated Monthly Payment After Residency	Interest Cost	Total Repayment
$0	Standard, but repay in five years via increased monthly payment	5	$5,100	$105,000	$305,000
$0	Standard	10	$2,900	$148,000	$348,000
$0	Extended	25	$1,700	$299,000	$499,000
$0	PAYE and REPAYE	13.2	$2,100 to $2,900	$185,000	$385,000

*When sending additional payments, the maximum monthly payment reached may be lower than expected (when simply adding the additional payment to the first row's maximum) because the loans will be paid off before reaching that maximum level.

Note: Values for repayment years and dollar amounts were rounded and are based on a 0% interest from March 13, 2020, through Jan. 31, 2022. Payments during residency are based on an average resident's stipend and a family size of one.

Use the MedLoans Organizer and Calculator to see the full impact of these repayment options on your loan portfolio.

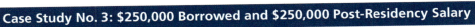

Case Study No. 3: $250,000 Borrowed and $250,000 Post-Residency Salary

PAYE Payments During a Four-Year Residency

Monthly Payment During Residency	Repayment Plan: **PAYE**	Repayment Years After Residency	Estimated Monthly Payment After Residency	Interest Cost	Total Repayment	Taxable Forgiveness (after 20 Years in PAYE)
$330 to $410	During and after residency	16	$2,100 to $3,000	$253,000	$503,000	≈$14,000
$330 to $410	During residency, then Standard	6	$5,200	$144,000	$394,000	$0
$330 to $410	During and after residency + additional $500/mo after residency	12.9	$2,600 to $3,300	$221,000	$447,000	$0
$330 to $410	During and after residency + additional $1,000/mo after residency	10.6	$3,100 to 3,700	$192,000	$442,000	$0

REPAYE Payments During a Four-Year Residency

Monthly Payment During Residency	Repayment Plan: **REPAYE**	Repayment Years After Residency	Estimated Monthly Payment After Residency	Interest Cost	Total Repayment	Taxable Forgiveness (after 25 Years in REPAYE)
$330 to $410	During and after residency	15.1	$2,100 to $3,000	$220,000	$470,000	$0
$330 to $410	During residency then Standard	6	$4,800	$16,000	$366,000	$0
$330 to $410	During and after residency + additional $500/mo after residency*	11.8	$2,600 to $3,200	$179,000	$429,000	$0
$330 to $410	During and after residency + additional $1,000/mo after residency*	9.7	$3,100 to $3,600	$155,000	$405,000	$0

Forbearance During a Four-Year Residency

Monthly Payment During Residency	Repayment Plan	Repayment Years After Residency	Estimated Monthly Payment After Residency	Interest Cost	Total Repayment	Taxable Forgiveness
$0	Standard, but repay in five years via increased monthly payment	5	$6,400	$136,000	$386,000	$0
$0	Standard	10	$3,700	$193,000	$443,000	$0
$0	Extended	25	$2,100	$389,000	$639,000	$0
$0	PAYE & REPAYE	18.1	$2,100 to $3,300	$314,000	$564,000	$0

*When sending additional payments, the maximum monthly payment reached may be lower than expected (when simply adding the additional payment to the first row's maximum) because the loans will be paid off before reaching that maximum level.

Note: Values for repayment years and dollar amounts were rounded and are based on a 0% interest from March 13, 2020, through Jan. 31, 2022. Payments during residency are based on an average resident's stipend and a family size of one.

Use the MedLoans Organizer and Calculator to see the full impact of these repayment options on your loan portfolio.

aamc.org/FIRST

Case Study No. 4: Borrowed $300,000 and $250,000 Post-Residency Salary

PAYE Payments During a Four-Year Residency

Monthly Payment During Residency	Repayment Plan: PAYE	Repayment Years After Residency	Estimated Monthly Payment After Residency	Interest Cost	Total Repayment	Taxable Forgiveness (after 20 Years in PAYE)
$330 to $410	During and after residency	16	$2,100 to $3,000	$204,000	$504,000	≈180,000
$330 to $410	During residency then Standard	6	$6,400	$177,000	$477,000	$0
$330 to $410	During and after residency + additional $500/mo after residency	16	$2,600 to $3,500	$300,000	$600,000	≈33,000
$330 to $410	During and after residency + additional $1,000/mo after residency*	13.7	$3,100 to $3,900	$282,000	$582,000	$0

REPAYE Payments During a Four-Year Residency

Monthly Payment During Residency	Repayment Plan: REPAYE	Repayment Years After Residency	Estimated Monthly Payment After Residency	Interest Cost	Total Repayment	Taxable Forgiveness (after 25 Years in REPAYE)
$330 to $410	During and after residency	19.7	$2,100 to $3,400	$345,000	$645,000	$0
$330 to $410	During residency then Standard	6	$5,900	$141,000	$441,000	$0
$330 to $410	During and after residency + additional $500/mo after residency*	15.3	$2,600 to $3,500	$270,000	$570,000	$0
$330 to $410	During and after residency + additional $1,000/mo after residency*	12.4	$3,100 to $3,800	$226,000	$526,000	$0

Forbearance During a Four-Year Residency

Monthly Payment During Residency	Repayment Plan	Repayment Years After Residency	Estimated Monthly Payment After Residency	Interest Cost	Total Repayment	Taxable Forgiveness
$0	Standard, but repay in five years via increased monthly payment	5	$7,800	$167,000	$472,000	$0
$0	Standard	10	$4,500	$237,000	$544,000	$0
$0	Extended	25	$2,600	$479,000	$797,000	$0
$0	PAYE	20	$2,100 to $3,400	$341,000	$641,000	≈$158,000
$0	REPAYE	24.3	$2,100 to $3,800	$520,000	$820,000	≈$0

*When sending additional payments, the maximum monthly payment reached may be lower than expected (when simply adding the additional payment to the first row's maximum) because the loans will be paid off before reaching that maximum level.

Note: Values for repayment years and dollar amounts were rounded and are based on a 0% interest from March 13, 2020, through Jan. 31, 2022. Payments during residency are based on an average resident's stipend and a family size of one.

Use the MedLoans Organizer and Calculator to see the full impact of these repayment options on your loan portfolio.

Living on a Resident Stipend of $59,700*

YOU CAN AFFORD A STUDENT LOAN PAYMENT

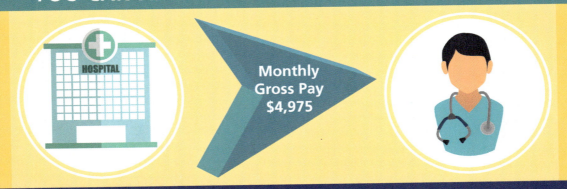

Monthly Gross Pay $4,975

WHAT HAPPENS TO YOUR PAYCHECK?

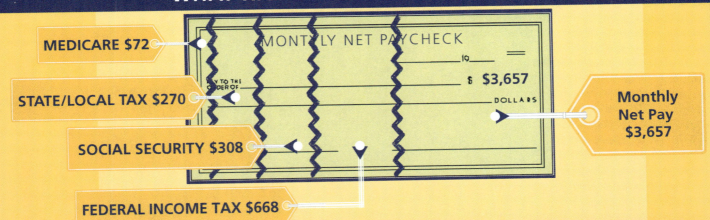

MONTHLY NET PAYCHECK

MEDICARE $72

STATE/LOCAL TAX $270

SOCIAL SECURITY $308

FEDERAL INCOME TAX $668

$ **$3,657**

DOLLARS

Monthly Net Pay $3,657

PAYMENTS ARE POSSIBLE ON A RESIDENT'S BUDGET

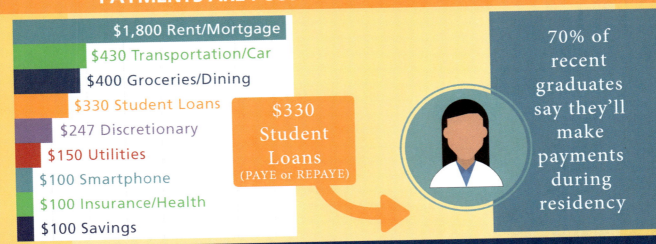

$1,800 Rent/Mortgage
$430 Transportation/Car
$400 Groceries/Dining
$330 Student Loans
$247 Discretionary
$150 Utilities
$100 Smartphone
$100 Insurance/Health
$100 Savings

$330 Student Loans
(PAYE or REPAYE)

70% of recent graduates say they'll make payments during residency

Based on a projected 2022 resident stipend. Paycheck breakdown and budgeted living costs are based on FIRST analysis of national averages.

aamc.org/FIRST

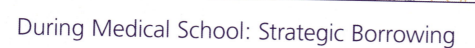

During Medical School: Strategic Borrowing

Options to Consider

For the majority of medical school students, borrowing student loans is a necessary component of completing a medical education. Despite this, it is important to know that there is a right way — and a wrong way — to get into debt. Understanding how to borrow strategically will enable you to borrow less, reduce your interest costs, and repay your student loans earlier.

Consideration No. 1: Alternatives to Borrowing

Borrowing wisely may mean not borrowing at all. There are other sources of monies that can reduce or eliminate the need to borrow. These alternatives include scholarships from outside sources such as faith-based groups, civic organizations, and state of residency. There are service-based scholarships such as military and public health service programs (e.g., National Health Service Corps). There may also be scholarships from your institution — check with the financial aid office for more details about those.

Don't forget family support — both financial and emotional. Whether parents, grandparents, or a working spouse, your family may be able to provide an alternative to borrowing. If, however, they are unable to contribute large gifts toward your education costs up front, family members are sometimes able to help pay the accruing interest on your student loans while you are in school. Such assistance can help reduce your repayment costs.

If you do not find alternatives to borrowing during medical school, familiarize yourself with **loan forgiveness and repayment options** available after graduation and during residency. The AAMC's website (aamc.org/stloan) lists many options for debt forgiveness and assistance. Remember, your **medical school's financial aid office** is your primary point of contact for all financial aid matters; visit it to discuss alternative sources of funding.

The Impact of the National Health Service Corps (NHSC) Loan Repayment

Primary care providers may receive substantial financial benefits by participating in either of the following programs.

NHSC Loan Repayment Program (NHSC LRP): For example, the minimum two-year commitment required of this program can result in a $50,000 award. If borrowers apply the entire award immediately to their outstanding balances, they would experience dramatic savings of time and money.

Medical school debt: **$200,000**

NHSC LRP applied post-residency: **$50,000***

Total repayment cost: **$263,000 over 15 years**

Total savings of NHSC LRP: **$110,000 and 4 years**

The impact of the NHSC LRP would be greater for higher debt levels.

*The award amount is based on the HPSA score of the site where the recipient works.

NHSC Student to Service Loan Repayment Program (S2S LRP): If borrowers apply their S2S award to their unpaid interest and principal, this larger award would lead to an even greater savings of time and money.

Medical school debt: **$200,000**

S2S LRP applied during residency: **$120,000**

Total repayment cost: **$172,000 over 11 years**

Total savings of S2S LRP: **$210,000 and 9 years**

The impact of the S2S LRP would be greater for higher debt levels.

Both NHSC scenarios are compared with a baseline scenario of a three-year residency program with Revised Pay As You Earn (REPAYE) during residency and a primary care position with a $190,000 salary after residency. This baseline results in a total repayment of $373,000 over 19 years.

For more information, refer to nhsc.hrsa.gov/loanrepayment.

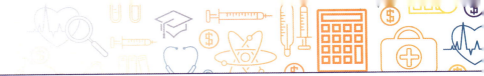

Consideration No. 2: Borrow in the Right Order

Borrowing wisely means borrowing the least expensive debt first and only considering more expensive student loans after your less costly options have been exhausted.

In the image to the right, the bottom tier translates into accepting all scholarships and grants (i.e., free money) before borrowing Primary Care Loans (PCL) and Loans for Disadvantaged Students (LDS), if eligible. After those options are exhausted, consider borrowing Direct Unsubsidized Loans, then Direct PLUS Loans, and, lastly, private loans or credit cards. If you choose a private loan, understand your options for repayment, deferment, and death or disability forgiveness because they may vary dramatically from those of federal student loans.

Your school and financial aid office have worked carefully to create a cost-of-attendance budget that, in most cases, limits excessive borrowing. Your award package is intended to enable you to avoid drastic financing options, such as private loans or credit cards. Contact your financial aid office to discuss your

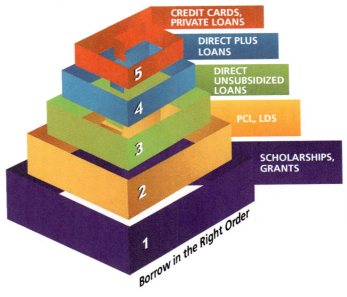

situation if you find yourself in the "red zone." Additionally, if an unexpected emergency occurs, your financial aid office may be able to assist in obtaining additional funds from sources other than private loans or credit cards. So, stay in touch with the office if a need arises.

Lastly, know that some schools may also offer **institutional loans**, which are loans lent directly by the school. These loans are not federal student loans, but they may come with enhanced borrower benefits such as lower interest rates, subsidies, and/or possible payment postponement or flexibility in repayment. Questions about institutional loans can be answered by your financial aid office. Also know that when you borrow certain loans, your eligibility for future aid may be affected. You are limited in the total amount of financial aid you receive each year, including all loans and scholarships. You are prohibited from receiving more aid than your cost of attendance. This could mean forfeiting free or lower-rate monies if you have already accepted a higher-rate loan — so always borrow in the right order.

Borrow smart. Maximize your least expensive debt first.

A Direct PLUS Loan at 6.28% can cost an additional $4,100 compared with a Direct Unsubsidized Loan. Borrowing $40,000 in private loans during medical school at 10.45% can cost an additional $23,700 compared with a Direct Unsubsidized Loan at 5.28%. Carefully consider all your loan options, and save money by borrowing wisely.

Note: The interest rate on private loans can vary according to market rates and a borrower's creditworthiness. Rates could be lower or higher than the rates used in this example, which assumes $10,000 in borrowing each year over four years, then a six-month grace period, and then a 10-year repayment term for each loan type.

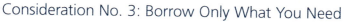

Consideration No. 3: Borrow Only What You Need

A common misconception that new medical school students have is that they are required to accept and borrow all the loans that are made available to them; however, this is not the case. The full amount that you are eligible to borrow does not have to be accepted up front. Rather, you can elect to accept only the amount you actually need, DECLINE the rest, and, if an unexpected emergency or cost arises, you can work with the financial aid office to gain access to those previously declined monies. In this manner, you protect yourself from overborrowing and, thus, reduce the chance of increasing your costs unnecessarily.

When you avoid borrowing more than what you need, you protect yourself from:

1. Origination costs for the unneeded money.

2. Interest costs that would accrue on the balance of funds that weren't needed.

3. Effects of capitalization on that extra money.

4. The possibility that this excess money may actually go toward things that you **want** rather than things you **need.**

The good news is, if you realize AFTER your loan disbursements have been received that you over borrowed, there is a 120-day window to return funds. Work with your financial aid office to send the unnecessary monies back to the loan servicer. This return of funds will reduce the principal balance you owe, as well as eliminate any origination fees or interest that may have accrued on the returned amount. On the other hand, if the window has closed and returning the extra monies is not an option, the financial aid office can help you offset this over borrowing by decreasing the amount of future disbursements.

COMMON MISTAKE: Hoping to be financially prepared for the coming semester/quarter, medical school students tend to think they should borrow everything that is made available to them.

CORRECT ACTION: Borrow only what you need and decline what you do not need. If additional monies are required in the future, the financial aid office can help you obtain the funds you previously declined.

CHALLENGE: Make a decision to borrow $5,000 less each year* than what is offered to you in your award package. If you choose to do this, you will avoid borrowing a total of $20,000 during medical school, which will result in reducing your:

Monthly Payment by roughly $322 per month

Total Interest Cost by $19,800

Make a plan — budget — and stick to it. Borrow only what you need to borrow because it will save you time and money during repayment.

*Example is based on a projected 2026 graduate borrowing federal loans (Direct Unsubsidized and Direct PLUS) at Congressional Budget Office projected interest rates with forbearance during a 3-year residency before beginning a 10-year Standard Repayment plan.

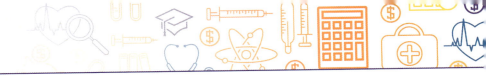

Consideration No. 4: Create a Budget

Have a plan. To successfully manage your financial life during medical school, you should have a plan, or budget, for how you will live on your borrowed money. Having this plan will help you not only know the amount you will need to live on — and thus, how much to borrow — it will also help you focus on spending your borrowed monies on things that you **need** (rather than things that you **want**). Remember, every dollar you spend while you are in medical school is a dollar that is likely accruing interest, and that interest may capitalize and then earn its own interest — making the cost of your medical school purchases ultimately far higher than you may anticipate.

> ### Live like a medical student while you are a medical student, and you will reap the rewards during repayment.

New medical school students, especially, may want to pay extra attention to the school's published cost of attendance (COA) and use it as a guide for determining how much may be needed to cover expenses in the first year. Many schools survey their students, so they know the cost of living in the area. The published COA is likely the best and most accurate estimate of current costs. So, start your medical education journey with a plan to determine:

- What you will need.
- How much you will borrow.
- How you will spend what you borrowed!

To reach your financial goals sooner, pay attention to the details of your financial life along the way.

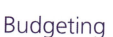

Budgeting

Having a spending plan is the cornerstone of a solid financial foundation. All other efforts for borrowing wisely or strategic repayment will be undermined if you don't have a plan of action for managing your finances. Living on a budget is possible, and by doing so, you will realize your financial goals sooner.

Benefits of Budgeting

Let's face it, money will probably be tight during residency. That's why having a realistic spending plan is essential for you to most efficiently accomplish the following:

- Track and control your spending.
- Identify leaks in your cash flow.
- Avoid credit card debt.
- Reduce your medical education debt.

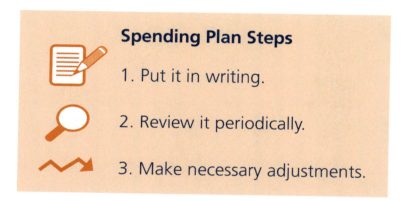

Creating a Budget

The most difficult part of developing a spending plan is taking the time to create it. This task may seem overwhelming at first, but it can be accomplished by using templates, guides, and other budgeting tools and websites. To get you started, the AAMC offers several tools to help create a budget, including budgeting worksheets for students and residents, articles, and ideas and tips. Visit aamc.org/FIRST.

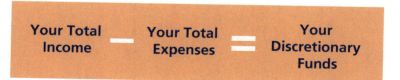

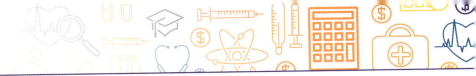

Basics of Budgeting

Income. The first step in creating a budget is to document all your incoming funds. If you are married, include your spouse's income as well. If you consistently receive gifts from family members, add these to your income. A refund check from the financial aid office also counts. Any incoming funds should be included in your income calculations.

Expenses. Next, identify all your monthly expenses, or monies, that are outgoing. There are two types of expenses, with the most obvious being routine, fixed amounts — including rent, car payments, insurance, and loans. Then, there are the expenses that fluctuate — such as clothing, gas, cell phone, groceries, and utilities. Total your monthly expenses, then subtract that amount from your income. What's left is the total of your discretionary funds.

Expenses

FIXED	VARIABLE
Rent	Groceries
Car payment	Entertainment
Insurance	Clothing
Student loan payment	Dining out
	Credit cards (debt)

Discretionary funds. Once all income has been determined and expenses have been honestly accounted for and properly subtracted, the remaining number is your bottom line (discretionary funds), the amount of leftover monies that may be used on the "extra" things in life such as entertainment, travel, and eating out. If you're being completely honest in your planning, you may find that your discretionary funds are a negative number. If so, go back and adjust until you break even.

On the other hand, if you have a positive bottom line that is significant (meaning there is a sizeable amount of money left over), you should perhaps run your numbers again. Have you accurately documented all your expenses? Typically, during residency, there won't be much extra money left over after your necessary expenses have been accounted for.

TIP: Choose to live like a student when you are a student so that you don't have to live like a student when you are a doctor, and likewise, live like a resident when you are a resident so you don't have to live like a resident after training is over. The AAMC's Financial Wellness program allows you to create a budget and track your expenses right from your phone or computer. Get started at aamc.org/financialwellness.

Finding Alternatives

Having a budget doesn't mean eliminating all the joy from your life; rather, it means keeping many of those "good" things and finding alternatives when necessary. Once your cash flow is visible in black and white, it will be easier to consciously reduce your cost of living. By periodically reviewing your budget for any imbalances, you'll realize that small adjustments can make a big difference.

Common alternatives for those living on a budget include:

- Buying groceries instead of eating out.
- Brewing your own coffee instead of going to a gourmet coffee shop.
- Choosing generic products instead of name brand.
- Opting for basic cable instead of a premium package or Netflix instead of the latest movies at a theater.
- Getting a roommate... or two instead of living alone.

Budget Worksheet for Students

For an interactive PDF of a student's budget, visit aamc.org/studentbudget.

MONTHLY INCOME:

Financial aid _____

Investment income _____

Gifts _____

Other _____

Total Monthly Income _____

MONTHLY FIXED EXPENSES:

Tuition and fees _____

Books and supplies _____

Savings _____

Rent/mortgage _____

Phone _____

Taxes (federal, state) _____

Vehicle payments _____

Other transportation _____

Personal loans _____

Education loans _____

Insurance (life and health) _____

Home/renter insurance _____

Auto insurance _____

Auto registration/taxes _____

Other _____

Total Fixed Expenses _____

MONTHLY VARIABLE EXPENSES:

Food/household supplies _____

Dining out _____

Clothes _____

Laundry/dry cleaning _____

Gas, oil, auto maintenance _____

Parking _____

Medical/dental/eye care _____

Entertainment _____

Travel/vacation _____

Utilities _____

Music/books/journals _____

Personal care _____

Subscriptions _____

Cable TV and internet _____

Credit card payments _____

Charity/contributions/gifts _____

Savings for interviews/relocation _____

Test prep course/materials _____

Exam/licensing fees _____

Other _____

Total Variable Expenses _____

Plus Total Fixed Expenses _____

Equals Total Monthly Expenses _____

Total Income _____

Less Total Expenses _____

Equals Total Discretionary Income (or Deficit) _____

Budget Worksheet for Residents

For an interactive PDF of a resident's budget, visit aamc.org/residentbudget. An infographic on the subject can also be found at aamc.org/residentstipend.

MONTHLY INCOME:

Salary (after deductions)	_____
Spouse salary (after deductions)	_____
Investment income	_____
Gifts	_____
Other	_____
Total Monthly Income	_____

MONTHLY FIXED EXPENSES:

Savings	_____
Rent/mortgage	_____
Phone	_____
Taxes (federal, state)	_____
Vehicle payments	_____
Other transportation	_____
Personal loans	_____
Education loans	_____
Insurance (life and health)	_____
Home/renter insurance	_____
Auto insurance	_____
Auto registration/taxes	_____
Other	_____
Total Fixed Expenses	_____

MONTHLY VARIABLE EXPENSES:

Food/household supplies	_____
Dining out	_____
Clothes	_____
Laundry/dry cleaning	_____
Gas, oil, auto maintenance	_____
Parking	_____
Medical/dental/eye care	_____
Entertainment	_____
Travel/vacation	_____
Utilities	_____
Music/books/journals	_____
Personal care	_____
Subscriptions	_____
Cable TV and internet	_____
Credit card payments	_____
Charity/contributions/gifts	_____
Savings for interviews/relocation	_____
Test prep course/materials	_____
Exam/licensing fees	_____
Other	_____
Total Variable Expenses	_____
Plus Total Fixed Expenses	_____
Equals Total Monthly Expenses	_____
Total Income	_____
Less Total Expenses	_____
Equals Total Discretionary Income (or Deficit)	_____

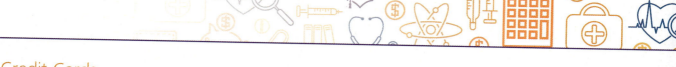

Credit Cards

Credit cards aren't bad; they have many positive financial aspects including the ability to use someone else's money for free for 30 days (depending on the terms of the card). Credit cards can also be used to improve your credit score by helping to establish a positive credit history when paid on time and not overused. Credit cards may also serve as a tool to track your spending and as a source of "rewards" for the purchases that you make, especially considering the rewards that could accumulate and be used for airfare, lodging, and other costs associated with residency interviews. Credit cards can also be helpful in emergencies. Despite these advantages, we are more familiar with the negative side of credit cards. What we hear about repeatedly is America's bad relationship with debt, which most often comes in the form of credit card debt. If used irresponsibly, credit cards will have a negative impact on your financial well-being.

> In the 2021 AAMC Graduation Questionnaire (GQ) survey, 14% of medical graduates reported having credit card debt, with a median amount of $4,000.

Signs You Could Be Heading for Trouble

These are tangible signs that either you're headed for trouble — or you're already there:

- Relying on credit cards to pay for the basics, such as food and utilities.
- Continually responding to offers to transfer balances from one card to another.
- Increasing your credit line or applying for new credit cards.
- Not maintaining a financial cushion for an unplanned expense.
- Making only minimum monthly payments.
- Ignoring credit card statements.
- Maxing out your credit cards.

Fixing the Problem

First and foremost: GET HELP. You don't have to face this alone. Credit card debt can get out of control, but there are ways to take back control. Depending on your situation, there may be a variety of solutions.

- Talk to the financial aid office staff. Often, they have dealt with similar situations and will be able to provide guidance.
- Go back to the basics and work on a budget. Determine how to start paying down your credit card balances.
- Call your credit card companies to work out a repayment plan.
- Negotiate! You can often negotiate a better rate, especially if you've been a good customer. Educate yourself using resources provided by the Federal Trade Commission (FTC): consumer.ftc.gov/topics/dealing-debt.

If your situation is more complicated, seek the advice of a professional credit counselor.

Creditors would rather work with you than have you default on your debt.

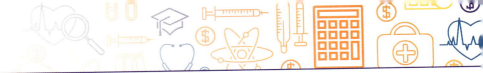

THE MINIMUM PAYMENT TRAP

$5,000 @ 18%
$5,000 financed at 18%

23 Years
Paying the minimum monthly payment means it will take you almost 23 years to fully repay.

$12,000 Total Paid
Paying the minimum monthly payment means you will pay $7,000 in interest.

What could possibly be worth paying more than twice its original value?

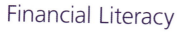

Financial Literacy

Identity Theft

In 2020, identity fraud in the United States cost victims $56 billion in total, with **traditional identity theft** accounting for $13 billion in losses (a 21% decrease from 2019), while **identity fraud scams** dramatically increased (due to the pandemic) and robbed victims of $43 billion. The facts below reflect a significant risk for consumers, especially students. The key to prevention is education and awareness. If you think you may be a victim, contact the FTC at identitytheft.gov. Don't become a statistic!

Friendly fraud
(when the perpetrator knows the victim) doubled last year for 25- to 34-year-olds.

Identity fraud scams:
Criminals directly contact and entrap the victim. Consumers often know (in hindsight) exactly when they were scammed.

One in 5 who experience identity theft will be victims of identity theft again.

68% of people reveal their birth date on a social networking site.

Traditional identity theft:
Criminals defeat an institution's fraud prevention technology, so consumers often don't know when or how they became victims.

87% of people leave personal information exposed.

LinkedIn, Google+, Twitter, and Facebook users are **more likely** to be victims.

In 2020, there were **1,387,615** identity theft reports in the U.S.

38-48% of victims discover their identities were stolen **within 3 months**.

Studies show that people earning **more than $75,000** have a greater chance of having their identity stolen.

26% of all complaints to the FTC concerning identity theft came from people ages 30 to 39.

One out of every 15 people are victims of identity fraud in the U.S.

Mobile account takeover **increased 78%** in 2018.

Smartphone users are **one-third** more likely to become a victim.

Sources: *Federal Trade Commission, 2016-2021; Javelin Strategy and Research, 2011-2021; Review42.com, 2021; Bureau of Justice Statistics,* Victims of Identity Theft, *2016.*

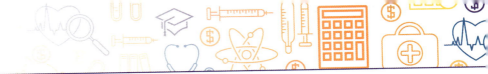

Stay Safe Online

- Turn on two-factor authentication wherever possible.
- Secure your devices (via a screen lock and encrypting data stored on the device).
- Avoid connecting to public Wi-Fi.
- Check your credit report (annualcreditreport.com).
- Install and update firewalls, antivirus software, and antispyware.
- Use and recognize secure websites.
- Avoid accessing personal accounts or sharing personal information (credit and debit cards) on:
  - Public computers.
  - Unsecured Wi-Fi connections (if a connection is unavoidable).
- Watch out for emails and attachments from imitators (banks, government, etc.).
- Use safe passwords.
  - Do not use the word "password."
  - Integrate numbers and symbols into your password.
  - Make your password at least eight characters long.

Stay Safe Offline

- Place a security freeze on your credit report.
- Request alerts on your accounts.
- Check your credit report at least annually.
- Consider credit monitoring or identity theft insurance.
- Keep personal documents, at home and work, safe and out of sight.
- Avoid sharing your Social Security number.
- Ask for an alternative identifier unrelated to your Social Security number.
- Carry only necessary documents and cards with you.
- Shred all documents with sensitive information.
- Request electronic statements.
- Use online bill pay.
- Opt out of preapproved credit card offers (optoutprescreen.com).
- Enter your debit card PIN discreetly.
- Be aware of your surroundings at all times.
- Pay attention to breach-notification letters — one in four breaches results in identity theft.

Be Social. Be Responsible.

There are a number of precautions to take when using social media. Here are just a few tips.

Be careful when revealing personal information on social media sites. Potential hackers could search your postings for details such as your date of birth, pets' names, and high school name and then use that information to change the password on your account. Hackers who can answer a security question with your personal information can then change your password and gain access to your account.

Use caution with social networking applications. Some applications may access your private information if it's not secure.

Be selective in choosing people to communicate with on social media sites. If you don't know the person requesting communication, don't accept the invitation.

Assume everything you post is permanent. Everyone wants to share good times and special events, but think about who may view a photo or something you said that could be taken as irresponsible or unprofessional.

Credit

Your Credit Score: What It Is and Why It Matters

A credit score is an indicator of the creditworthiness of an individual. In other words, it is a numerical value that represents the probability that a borrower will repay a debt. This score is important because it will directly affect your approval rate (for insurance, housing, utilities, and more) and your interest rate for loans. In most situations, the better your credit score, the less it will cost you to borrow.

During residency, focusing on the following items will improve your credit score:

1. Pay your bills on time.

2. Pay down your debt. Limit the amount of debt you put on credit cards (revolving lines of credit).

3. Don't close accounts, and do limit opening new ones.

After four or more years of watching and protecting your credit, it's possible that you'll have a better credit score than when you started medical school.

How Your Credit Score Is Determined

A credit score is based on the content of your credit report. The best known and most commonly used credit score is a FICO Score, with values ranging from 300 to 850. Knowing your exact FICO Score is not as important as understanding what determines this number.

Nothing in Life Is Free, Right?

If you want to know your credit score, there are numerous ways to get it for free. It may be offered as a benefit from your bank or credit card or even from one of the many credit score monitoring agencies (like creditkarma.com, creditsesame.com, or bankrate.com/quizzle). Many of these sources allow you to see your score for free and explain your score by highlighting areas for improvement. However, keep in mind that after using free services, you will likely be marketed to by the agency or their partner companies. Choose the source of your score analysis carefully, always read the fine print, and reveal your personal information only to sources you trust. Time is better spent reviewing your credit report, which you can do here: annualcreditreport.com. (Where it really is free!)

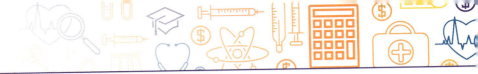

Breakdown of a FICO Score

A credit score, or FICO Score, is based on five factors, none of which considers employment status, income, or profession. Be aware of these factors because even though you will be an MD, a good credit score is not guaranteed.

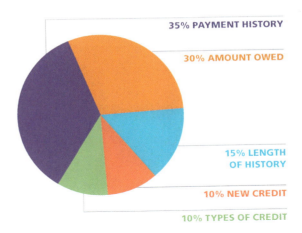

35% PAYMENT HISTORY

30% AMOUNT OWED

15% LENGTH OF HISTORY

10% NEW CREDIT

10% TYPES OF CREDIT

Payment History (35%)

This is the largest portion of your score. Delinquent payments can have a negative impact on scoring, but consistent on-time payments will raise a credit score.

TIP: As a resident, be proactive about paying on time. Set up automatic withdrawal, or schedule online bill-pay services with your bank so that a recurring monthly payment (such as for a credit card) is never late.

Amount Owed (30%)

The total amount of the credit line that you are currently using will affect your credit score. The goal is to use less than 30% of your line of credit (add up the maximum credit line on all your credit cards and multiply by 0.30 to determine the goal for your utilization rate).

TIP: During residency, make a focused effort to pay down your credit card debt or, at a minimum, avoid increasing the balance on these cards.

Length of History (15%)

The longer the history, the higher the score, so avoid starting new lines of credit. The length of your credit history is determined by calculating the average age of all your lines of credit; new lines of credit will reduce this average.

TIP: Avoid opening new lines of credit and take care of your old lines of credit (do not close them if you don't have to). Closed accounts eventually fall off your report, and this could hurt your history.

New Credit (10%)

Even a single new line of credit can hurt your score, but a lot of inquiries from lenders viewing your credit report, because of your requests for new lines of credit, can cause a double-digit drop. Only request new lines of credit when it's absolutely necessary.

TIP: When you're checking out at your favorite store, if the salesperson asks if you would like to apply for the store credit card, just say no.

Types of Credit (10%)

Having a variety of types of credit (e.g., a mortgage, credit cards, student loans, car loan) is good for your credit score.

TIP: Having too much of one thing — such as lines of revolving credit (e.g., credit cards) — is never good for your credit, so be aware of how many credit cards you have. For more information, visit myfico.com.

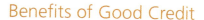

Benefits of Good Credit

Good credit means you are more likely to get a loan approved. Beyond that, you'll enjoy:

- Better loan offers (rates, terms, and conditions).
- Lower interest rates on credit cards.
- Faster credit approvals.
- Increased leasing and rental options.
- Reduced security deposits.
- Reduced premiums on auto, home, renter, and life insurance policies.

Being proactive about your credit is the way to begin making smart financial decisions that will give you a solid financial foundation for years to come.

Credit Reports

You have three credit reports. A separate credit report is maintained by each of the three major credit reporting agencies — Equifax, Experian, and TransUnion. These three reports accomplish the same purpose, but the information on each report may vary. To protect yourself from mistakes and identity theft, you should review each of your credit reports annually.

Reality Check: Scrutinize Your Credit Report

It is a good idea to review your credit report at least once a year. You can request a copy of your free report from each of the three major credit bureaus online. To order your free report, visit annualcreditreport.com. Normally, you are entitled to a free report from each credit bureau once a year, but due to the increased identity theft attempts that occurred during the pandemic, at this time **consumers can access their free credit report on a weekly basis** — so take advantage of this now and in the future!

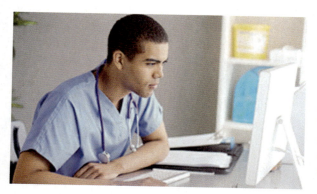

Financial Wellness for Medical School and Beyond

The AAMC wants to provide you with practical information that can help you with budgeting, money management, credit, debt management, and more. With the AAMC Financial Wellness program, you can access articles, interactive exercises, and a curriculum covering a multitude of financial topics. To get started, visit aamc.org/financialwellness.

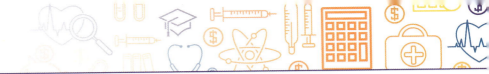

Other Considerations

Public Service Loan Forgiveness (PSLF)

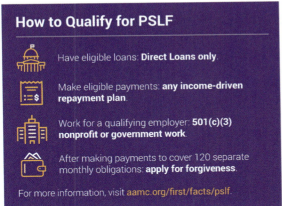

How to Qualify for PSLF

Have eligible loans: **Direct Loans only**.

Make eligible payments: **any income-driven repayment plan**.

Work for a qualifying employer: **501(c)(3) nonprofit or government work**.

After making payments to cover 120 separate monthly obligations: **apply for forgiveness**.

For more information, visit aamc.org/first/facts/pslf.

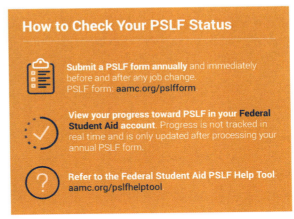

How to Check Your PSLF Status

Submit a PSLF form annually and immediately before and after any job change. PSLF form: aamc.org/pslfform

View your progress toward PSLF in your Federal Student Aid account. Progress is not tracked in real time and is only updated after processing your annual PSLF form.

Refer to the Federal Student Aid PSLF Help Tool: aamc.org/pslfhelptool

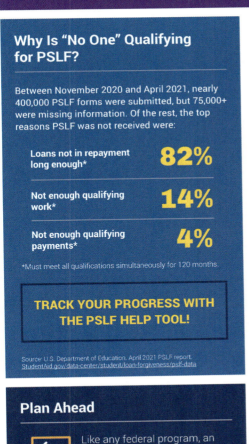

Why Is "No One" Qualifying for PSLF?

Between November 2020 and April 2021, nearly 400,000 PSLF forms were submitted, but 75,000+ were missing information. Of the rest, the top reasons PSLF was not received were:

Loans not in repayment long enough*	**82%**
Not enough qualifying work*	**14%**
Not enough qualifying payments*	**4%**

*Must meet all qualifications simultaneously for 120 months.

TRACK YOUR PROGRESS WITH THE PSLF HELP TOOL!

Source: U.S. Department of Education. April 2021 PSLF report. StudentAid.gov/data-center/student/loan-forgiveness/pslf-data

Plan Ahead

Like any federal program, an act of Congress could change PSLF, so **have a backup plan** for managing your student loan debt.

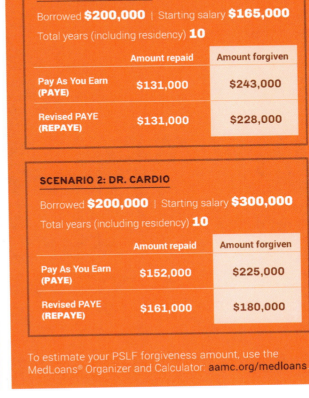

The Value of PSLF to a Physician

The forgiven amount has no limit and is not taxed.

SCENARIO 1: DR. PEDS

Borrowed **$200,000** | Starting salary **$165,000**

Total years (including residency) **10**

	Amount repaid	Amount forgiven
Pay As You Earn (PAYE)	$131,000	$243,000
Revised PAYE (REPAYE)	$131,000	$228,000

SCENARIO 2: DR. CARDIO

Borrowed **$200,000** | Starting salary **$300,000**

Total years (including residency) **10**

	Amount repaid	Amount forgiven
Pay As You Earn (PAYE)	$152,000	$225,000
Revised PAYE (REPAYE)	$161,000	$180,000

To estimate your PSLF forgiveness amount, use the MedLoans® Organizer and Calculator: aamc.org/medloans

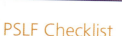

PSLF Checklist

If you decide to work in public service, you may be eligible for federal student loan forgiveness after 10 years of full-time work. The information below outlines the qualifying components of the PSLF program, and a timeline of action to enter PSLF is included on page 58.

This checklist is a general guideline only. For more information, watch a FIRST video on pursuing PSLF at aamc.org/first/pslfguide. You can also read more about PSLF on the FSA website or use the Department of Education's PSLF Help Tool at aamc.org/pslfhelptool to receive personalized guidance in your pursuit of PSLF.

Five steps to ensure eligibility for Public Service Loan Forgiveness

Step 1: Request a qualifying repayment plan for your eligible loans (recertify annually).
Step 2: If necessary, consolidate eligible FFEL, LDS, and Perkins Loans into a Direct Consolidation Loan.
Step 3: To verify employment eligibility, submit the PSLF form via the PSLF Help Tool and resubmit it annually.
Step 4: Make 120 qualifying payments while completing eligible work.
Step 5: Upon completion of requirements, complete the PSLF form to apply for forgiveness.

Checklist for Public Service Loan Forgiveness

☐ **ELIGIBLE LOANS** Only the following loan types are eligible:

- Direct Loans (Subsidized and Unsubsidized)
- Direct PLUS and parent PLUS Loans
- Direct Consolidation Loans
- Other federal student loans* can be made eligible by including them in a Direct Consolidation Loan.**

*FFEL Stafford, Grad PLUS, federal consolidation, Perkins, LDS, and certain other FFEL loans.
**More information is available at StudentAid.gov.
NOTE: Defaulted loans, private loans, and any consolidation loan containing a spousal consolidation loan are not eligible.

☐ **QUALIFYING PAYMENTS** While simultaneously working in a qualifying public service position, you must make 120 on-time and scheduled payments* under a qualifying repayment plan. The following plans qualify:

- Income-Based Repayment (IBR)
- Pay As You Earn (PAYE)
- Revised Pay As You Earn (REPAYE)
- Income-Contingent Repayment (ICR)

- Standard Repayment plan (or a repayment plan where the monthly amount paid is not less than the monthly amount required under the 10-year Standard Repayment plan)

*Payments do not have to be consecutive, allowing for changes in employers and periods of nonwork.

☐ **QUALIFYING WORK** You must be employed full-time* for a total of 10 years in a public service position. For the work to be considered public service, your employer must be one of the following:

- Nonprofit tax-exempt 501(c)(3) organization (includes many medical schools and residency programs)
- Federal, state, local, or tribal government organization, agency, or entity
- A branch of the military
- Public service organization — a private organization providing a public service

*Full-time work is considered to be 30 hours per week or the number of hours the employer considers to be full-time.

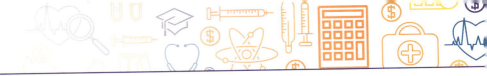

Action Plan: Entering PSLF

For Every PSLF Applicant

Action 1: Plan to request the income-driven repayment (IDR) plan that offers you the lowest monthly payment. Keep in mind, the PAYE plan offers a capped payment amount, and compared to the other plans, this could help minimize your overall cost while pursuing PSLF. You can request any IDR plan online at StudentAid.gov about 90 days before the end of your grace period. Check with your loan servicer to verify when they will accept an IDR request.

If You Have FFEL or Perkins Loans *(or want to enter repayment immediately)*

Action 2: If you have FFEL or Perkins loans and you want them to qualify for forgiveness through PSLF, then you must consolidate them to make them eligible. After separating from medical school, **apply to consolidate these loans** and have them put into a Direct Consolidation Loan* — you can do this in your FSA account (StudentAid.gov). As you complete the consolidation application, be sure to indicate:

- Your interest in PSLF.
- An IDR plan to pay the consolidation loan under.
- The timeframe to begin processing your application.

Keep in mind that Direct Loans do not need to be consolidated; a Direct Loan is eligible for PSLF as-is, but consolidating any federal loan will eliminate the existing grace period, causing loans to enter repayment as soon as the application is processed. If the application is processed immediately after graduating, entry into a PSLF qualifying repayment plan could occur earlier than if the full grace period had been experienced.

If you need to consolidate but also want to experience your full grace period, then request processing to begin a month or two before the grace is over (so payments won't be due until after the consolidation has been disbursed). Processing of a consolidation takes 30-75 days. Payments made toward the consolidation loan must be under a qualifying repayment plan (refer to page 56 for a list of these plans).

For Every PSLF Applicant

Action 3: When you begin work in your residency program, you should submit a PSLF form so your employer's eligibility can be verified and your progress toward PSLF can be tracked (aamc.org/PSLFform).

Action 4: Work toward PSLF by making your required payments. It is highly recommended you track your PSLF progress through the PSLF Help Tool. Borrowers can enroll in direct debit to ensure on-time payments (aamc.org/PSLFhelptool).

Action 5 (and on): Each year, you will need to update your income information and family size so the servicer can accurately calculate future monthly payments. Also, it is highly recommended that you submit the PSLF form annually, as well as immediately before and after any job change.

*Not all schools report a graduate's separation date immediately upon graduation. For this reason, your servicer may continue to view you as an enrolled student for weeks after graduation, meaning they won't be able to process your consolidation application until your enrollment status is updated.

The PSLF Limited Waiver

A **PSLF waiver** is now available for a limited time. On Oct. 6, 2021, the U.S. Department of Education relaxed regulations for PSLF to make it easier to obtain forgiveness under the PSLF program. The changes made most directly benefit federal student loan borrowers who have worked for a qualifying employer anytime since 2007 and have older student loans, referred to as FFELP loans. Learn more about this PSLF waiver opportunity at StudentAid.gov/PSLFWaiver.

Loan Consolidation

Consolidation of federal loans allows you to combine one or more existing federal student loans into a single loan. A consolidation loan pays off the old loans and gives you a single new loan with new terms, conditions, and a new interest rate. The advantages and disadvantages of consolidating depend on what loans you include in the consolidation and when you consolidate. To consolidate your federal student loans into a federal consolidation loan, visit StudentAid.gov.

Advantages	Disadvantages
• A single payment to a single servicer. • Possible lower monthly payment. • Extended repayment period. • No prepayment penalty. • Ability to change repayment plans. • Possible eligibility for PSLF. • Possible eligibility for an income-driven repayment plan. • Possible acceleration of repayment start date by forfeiture of grace time.	• Possibly longer repayment period resulting in higher interest costs. • Possible loss of current borrower benefits. • Possible disqualification of previously eligible PSLF payments. • Higher interest rate (interest rate is the weighted average of the loans rounded up to the nearest one-eighth of a percent). • Possible negative effect on grace, deferment, or forgiveness options.

For many medical students leaving school, the primary reason to consolidate is to simplify the repayment process during residency. This is especially true when multiple payments are required. Alternatively, if you would prefer to avoid consolidation, scheduling automatic payments from your bank account can simplify repayment (and eliminate the need to consolidate). Use the information on pages 61-62 to help determine if consolidation is right for you. **Borrowers enrolled in school are not eligible to consolidate.**

When Can I Start My Consolidation?

This question is often asked by those approaching graduation, and unfortunately, the answer is not as easy as it should be because it depends. **When you are able to initiate a federal loan consolidation depends on when your school reports you as being separated from school.** Some school systems report a separation date for all students (undergraduate, graduate, medical, etc.) that is much later than the date the medical students actually graduate. If you want to be certain about when you can consolidate your loans, find out when your school will report you as graduated or separated — often the registrar will know. Only after your servicer updates your loans with that date can your application for a Direct Consolidation loan be processed.

Reality Check: Consolidation May Mean Paying More Interest

It's important to realize that although loan consolidation can give you a lower monthly payment with a longer repayment term, this longer term can significantly increase the total cost of the debt.

The longer you take to repay a loan, the more it will cost because interest is accruing for a longer period of time. Also, most of your federal loans already have fixed interest rates, meaning that consolidation could result in a slightly higher fixed interest rate (due to rounding).

Understand how consolidation works before consolidating — in most cases, it is permanent.

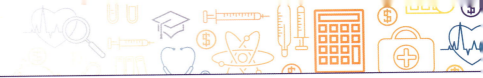

Effects of Student Loan Consolidation

Loan Type	Simplify Repayment[1]	Lower Monthly Payment[2]	Make Eligible for PSLF/PAYE/REPAYE[3]	Forfeit Grace Period[4]	Fix a Variable Rate[5]	Make Eligible for Residency Forbearance or IBR[6]	Loss of Interest Subsidy[7]	Grace and Deferment Options Lost[8]
Direct Subsidized Loans	X	X		X	X			
Direct Unsubsidized Loans	X	X		X	X			
Federal Subsidized Stafford Loans	X	X	X	X	X			
Federal Unsubsidized Stafford Loans	X	X	X	X	X			
Direct PLUS Loans	X	X		X				
Grad PLUS Loans	X	X	X	X				
Perkins Loans	X	X	X	X		X	X	X
LDS Loans	X	X	X	X		X	X	X
Direct Consolidation Loans	X	X						
Federal Consolidation Loans	X	X	X					

■ = Benefits
■ = Consequences

1. **Simplify Repayment.** The main benefit of loan consolidation for medical residents is simplification of the repayment process by combining all federal student loans into a single new loan with one point of contact and a single required monthly payment. This is a valuable benefit for those who have little time or energy to manage personal financial matters.

2. **Lower Monthly Payment.** Before consolidating, most loans have a 10-25-year repayment term, but after consolidating, the loan term is lengthened up to 30 years. This longer term causes the required monthly payment to decrease significantly — a great benefit if cash flow is limited. On the other hand, an extended term can also mean higher interest costs. The good news is that there is no prepayment penalty for federal loans, so extra payments are allowed and encouraged at any time to reduce the total interest cost.

3. **Make Eligible for PSLF/PAYE/REPAYE.** Loans that were not originally disbursed from Direct Loans are not eligible for Public Service Loan Forgiveness (PSLF) or the Pay As You Earn (PAYE) and Revised Pay As You Earn (REPAYE) repayment plans. However, if eligible federal student loans (Perkins Loans, for example) are included in a Direct Consolidation Loan, they become eligible for PSLF and the PAYE and REPAYE repayment plans. Other eligibility requirements also need to be met.

4. **Forfeit Grace Period.** Consolidation loans do not have a grace period, and monthly payments will be required within 60 days of the consolidation loan being disbursed. For this reason, if you want to use your entire grace period, you will need to either 1) request that the servicer delay the processing of the consolidation until the end or near the end of the grace period (this request is made in the consolidation application) OR 2) wait to complete a consolidation application until after all grace periods have been fully exhausted. On the other hand, consolidation is the only way to "skip" the grace period — call it an unintended loophole. Borrowers seeking loan forgiveness may want to start making payments immediately after graduation because the sooner payments begin, the earlier forgiveness can be obtained in a number of programs; consolidation will accelerate the start time of these payments by "skipping" the grace period.

   Direct PLUS Loans do not have a grace period; however, they do have a post-enrollment deferment that behaves much like a grace period (postponing payments) and lasts for six months. This deferment occurs automatically and is lost if the Direct PLUS Loans are consolidated before the entire six months of post-enrollment deferment have occurred.

5. **Fix a Variable Rate.** (This benefit is applicable only to loans disbursed before July 1, 2006.) The interest rate on a consolidation loan is based on the weighted average of the underlying loans, rounded up to the nearest one-eighth of a percent, and then fixed for the life of the loan. A fixed rate is protected from rate changes and may be financially worthwhile for variable rate loans. However, very few medical graduates have these older variable rate student loans; therefore, the effect of consolidation on fixed interest rate loans is likely to be an increase in the interest rate because of the rounding process.

6. **Make Eligible for Residency Forbearance or IBR.** Perkins Loans and LDS Loans are not eligible for Mandatory Medical Residency Forbearance or the Income-Based Repayment (IBR) plan in their original form. These loans, however, can be included in a Direct Consolidation Loan, making the debt eligible to be postponed with a resident forbearance or repaid under IBR. All other federal student loans are eligible for repayment under IBR in their original form and with their current servicer. (Note: Parent PLUS Loans are not eligible for IBR.)

7. **Loss of Interest Subsidy.** In their original form, Perkins and LDS Loans are subsidized, which means that interest does not accrue while the loan is in an in-school, grace, or deferment status. When a Perkins or LDS Loan is consolidated, the balance of the loan becomes unsubsidized.

8. **Grace and Deferment Options Lost.** Certain loans are eligible for additional time in grace or deferment, but when these loans are consolidated, the remaining balance on these loans loses these options.

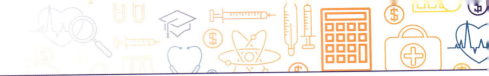

Should You Consider a Direct Loan Consolidation?

Are you wondering if consolidation is right for you? Answer these questions to find out.

1. Do you have multiple servicers for your federal student loans?

Yes, a consolidation with Direct Loans may offer you the much-needed benefit of simplification: one loan, one point of contact, and one payment. One of the top reasons medical residents consolidate is to simplify the management of their federal student loans during residency.

No, loan consolidation would not provide an obvious benefit in managing your loans.

2. Are you considering work in public service and Public Service Loan Forgiveness (PSLF)?

Yes, a Direct Consolidation Loan may be necessary to make some of your debt eligible for this forgiveness program. You would NOT need to include all your loans in the consolidation. Only the federal loans that do not already have the word "Direct" in their name would need to be consolidated since these are ineligible for PSLF in their current form. To find your federal student loans, log in to your FSA account at StudentAid.gov.

No, loan consolidation would not provide any obvious benefit based on your career goals.

Possibly. Refer to the advice for those who answered yes (to the left), and then strongly consider following it. This approach leaves your options open: In the future, you can choose between continuing on the path toward forgiveness under PSLF or leaving public service without penalty.

3. Would you benefit from a lower required monthly payment?

Yes, loan consolidation may benefit your monthly budget because it can dramatically reduce your required monthly payment. This is accomplished by stretching the term of the original loans from 10 years to up to 30 years. Keep in mind, the longer it takes to pay off a loan, the more the loan can cost. However, there are no prepayment penalties on federal student loans, so a consolidation loan can be paid off earlier than required by sending extra money when possible, which will help avoid the additional interest costs.

Alternatively, a lower monthly payment can be obtained without consolidating. By changing your selected repayment plan to an income-driven plan, you could qualify for an even lower monthly payment during residency — possibly making consolidation unnecessary. Discuss this option with your loan servicers.

No, loan consolidation would not provide an obvious benefit to your financial situation. By not consolidating, you avoid stretching out the term of the loan. Therefore, you'll probably repay the balance of your debt sooner, which will cost you less in interest.

Possibly. Refer to the advice for those who answered yes (to the left), and then strongly consider following it. This approach gives you the flexibility to pay less when you need to and more when you can.

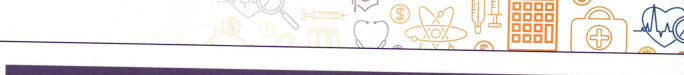

4. Do you have private student loans in addition to your federal student loans?

Yes, medical residents sometimes find it difficult to repay both private and federal loans — at least during residency. A helpful strategy may be to consolidate all federal loans, to obtain a single servicer (a benefit discussed in Question 1), and then to request a postponement of payment while in residency. Postponement is easily accomplished with a Mandatory Medical Residency Forbearance. Then, while payments on your federal loans are postponed, you can focus on the private debt and attempt to repay it in full, as soon as possible.

No, loan consolidation would not provide an obvious benefit in managing your loans.

5. Are you considering an income-driven repayment plan?

Yes, a Direct Consolidation may be needed to make some of your loans eligible for these repayment plans. Specifically, Perkins and LDS Loans are not eligible for income-driven repayment plans — so these loans would need to be consolidated to become eligible. Your federal student loans that do not have the word "Direct" in their name would need to be consolidated to gain eligibility for the PAYE/REPAYE repayment plans. For questions about eligibility, call your servicers.

No, loan consolidation would not provide an obvious benefit for your repayment plan options.

6. After graduating, do you want to start making required payments as soon as possible?

Yes, although there is no way to forfeit or skip the grace period on federal student loans; when these loans are included in a Direct Consolidation Loan, any existing grace periods are gone/lost/forfeited ... or "skipped" when the new consolidation loan is disbursed. Therefore, consolidation provides an unintended consequence that can benefit those seeking to begin repayment immediately (which may allow borrowers to obtain loan forgiveness four to six months earlier because the sooner you start making required payments, the earlier you may be able to reach forgiveness).

No, loan consolidation would not provide an obvious benefit to your financial situation. By not consolidating, you leave your grace period intact, allowing you the time you need to transition (financially and physically) out of medical school and into residency.

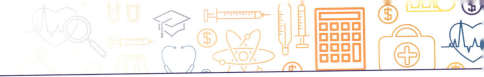

Student Loan Refinancing (Private Consolidation)

There are lenders that will refinance your federal student loans into a private loan, and though they may refer to this as a consolidation, there are significant differences between consolidating into a Direct Consolidation Loan and refinancing into a private loan. **If your federal loans are put into a private loan, you may lose all rights, terms, and conditions that are currently guaranteed to you — student loan tax deductions, discharge in case of death or disability, and forbearance while in residency, to name a few.** Additionally, most of the repayment options discussed in these pages are for federal loans but may not be an option for private loans. Prior to completing a consolidation or a refinance application, be sure you understand what you want to accomplish versus what your new loan will offer.

> For details on the repayment options for a private loan, contact the private loan lender.

Should I Refinance My Student Loans?

Answer these questions to find out.

If you have excellent credit, you may be able to refinance your existing **federal student loans** into a private loan to obtain more favorable interest rates. Before doing that, it's important to understand the full impact of making this permanent change to your loans.

1. Will this new private loan have a variable interest rate?

 Yes

Yes, if you refinance into a private loan with a low variable rate today, over time, the rate could rise higher than the current fixed rate on your federal loans. Variable rates are tied to an index causing the rate to rise or fall, which makes the total cost of variable rate debt impossible to calculate. Choosing variable rate loans involves taking some financial risk. Before committing to a variable rate loan, understand exactly how often the rate may change and how high it may rise. A variable rate loan could be a good option IF you will fully repay the loan in the near future.

 No

No, fixed rate loans offer stability to a borrower's repayment, making them a good option for borrowers who don't like risk. To make an accurate comparison of fixed rate private loans with other loans, be sure you know the terms, conditions, and fees (e.g., origination fees) of all the loans. **A fixed rate loan may be the best option if high levels of debt and long repayment terms are involved.**

2. Will you be working in public service? (This may include work during residency or a fellowship or while you are employed at an academic institution or at any level of the government.)

 Yes

Yes, after completing 10 years of public service work, as well as satisfying several other requirements, forgiveness may be granted on some or all of your remaining federal student loans. **Private loans are not eligible for Public Service Loan Forgiveness (PSLF). Only Direct Loans qualify for the PSLF program.**

 No

No, based on your expected career path, forfeiting access to Public Service Loan Forgiveness is not a factor you need to consider when deciding whether to refinance.

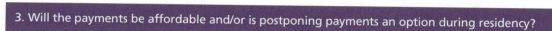

3. Will the payments be affordable and/or is postponing payments an option during residency?

Yes

No

Possibly

Yes, the lender determines the terms of private loans. If you cannot make your payments, you will be restricted to the accommodations offered by the private lender. However, with federal loans, a borrower has access to a variety of affordable payment plans and postponement options. For this reason, if you refinance with a private loan, select a reputable lender and thoroughly read the fine print.

No or not sure, repaying private student loans can be burdensome if you don't have access to the kind of flexible repayment and postponement options that federal student loans offer. So, know your current options in the federal program (such as income-driven repayment plans that limit the payment amounts and can lead to forgiveness or the ability to easily postpone payments during residency) and then question the private lender to see exactly how their terms and conditions compare. **In general, reputable lenders will warn you about the benefits you are giving up when refinancing federal student loans.**

4. Are you comfortable with assuming more risk in your financial life?

Refinancing with a private loan may be a good option if you are motivated to repay your student debt; have a secure job, emergency savings, and strong credit; are unlikely to benefit from forgiveness options; and have a low fixed rate option available OR you will have access to sufficient funds in the near future. However, if you do not meet these criteria, many financial advisors suggest that trading in federal loans for private loans will expose you to additional financial risk. Therefore, before you assume possible financial risk, evaluate your current situation to determine whether you could make it through if something unexpected occurs.

No matter what your future holds, federal student loans will give you the ability to benefit from their flexible terms and conditions, including access to income-driven repayment plans and possible loan forgiveness, potential interest subsidies, limits to monthly payment amounts, the availability of a death and disability discharge, and possible student loan tax deductions. Be sure the potential reward of a refinance is enough to offset the potential risk you will assume.

Private debt and federal debt can operate very differently, especially when it comes to repayment. Know what you're giving up and what you will gain because refinancing federal loans into a private loan cannot be undone.

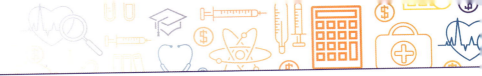

Debt Management Strategies for Private Loans

Two possible strategies to consider for repayment of private loans are detailed below.

Forbearance: A repayment strategy medical graduates who have both federal and private loans can use is to request a Mandatory Medical Residency Forbearance on their federal loans — causing the required payment on the federal loans to be zero. This postponement of payments for the federal loans allows aggressive payments to be made toward private debt. This strategy is most beneficial if the interest rates on the private loans are higher than the rates on the federal debt. Paying off loans with a high interest rate quickly is a wise strategy. However, interest rates aside, even if the rate of the private debt is not higher than that of the federal loans, the strategy of postponing federal payments may simply free up your cash flow and allow you to make your private loan's required monthly payments during residency.

Refinancing: Another repayment strategy is to refinance some or all of your private student debt. The first step to do this is to shop around for the loan with the best terms. You can start your search at your school's financial aid office. Your chance of obtaining a better interest rate on the new loan increases if your credit score has improved since you originally received the private loans or if you can get a creditworthy cosigner. However, the opposite is also true: A lower credit score may lead to higher interest costs. Also, be aware that if the refinanced loan offers a longer period of time for repayment, which will reduce the monthly payment, you will pay more in interest. Ideally, refinance into a loan that offers no prepayment penalty.

When you refinance to manage the repayment of private debt, the most important advice is to read the fine print for the loan, paying special attention to the terms, conditions, and costs of the new loan. Refinancing private debt has the potential to do more harm than good if it involves origination fees, increases your interest rate, or results in the loss of positive terms and conditions (aamc.org/first/shouldirefinance). So, proceed with caution.

> **Be sure to read all the fine print before signing.**

Borrower Benefits on Federal Student Loans

Good news: Your federal loans may have borrower benefits tied to them that can help you save time and money over the course of your repayment. These benefits are incentives, such as reduced interest rates, reimbursement of loan fees, or even getting money back. To obtain these benefits, you must perform a specific action, such as making uninterrupted, on-time payments or having funds automatically debited from your bank account. A common benefit available is a 0.25% interest rate reduction when you are signed up for automatic payment withdrawal. To find out what your benefits may be, contact your loan servicers. Also, be advised that existing borrower benefits could be permanently lost when you obtain a consolidation loan — so carefully consider your borrower benefits BEFORE consolidating.

Student Loan Interest — A Tax Deduction

More good news: The interest you pay on your student loans may be tax deductible (up to $2,500 annually). Certain parameters that must be met, though.

The maximum allowable deduction ($2,500) diminishes as your income increases according to your MAGI (modified adjusted gross income). This means that paying interest while in school and/or residency will not only help reduce capitalization and interest costs, it also could allow you to take advantage of a deduction that you may not qualify for in the future when your income increases.

	Full Deduction	Partial Deduction	No Deduction
Single	$70,000 or less	$70,001 to $84,999	$85,000 or more
Married filing jointly	$140,000 or less	$140,001 to $169,999	$170,000 or more

Source: IRS Publication 970, 2020.

For more detailed information, visit irs.gov and review IRS Publication 970, Tax Benefits for Higher Education.

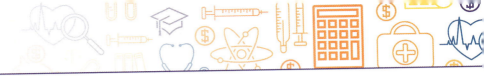

Lifetime Learning — A Tax Credit

A maximum of $2,000 in tax credits per year, called the Lifetime Learning Credit, is available for eligible students who have qualifying education expenses. As a credit, this tax benefit can only be used to reduce the amount of taxes owed and will not result in refundable cash if your income tax liability is less than $2,000. For more details about this tax credit and other possible tax benefits available to students, visit irs.gov and review IRS Publication 970, Tax Benefits for Higher Education.

Avoiding Delinquency and Default

Count yourself in good company: Default and delinquency rates among medical school borrowers are very low. Although low, they certainly are not zero. Usually, if borrowers run into difficulty during their residency years, it's because they don't keep in touch with their loan servicers or because they are late in filing deferment or forbearance forms. You have sacrificed too much and come too far to let this happen. Don't risk your financial future with carelessness — be organized about your repayment. Make sure you contact your servicers whenever your enrollment status, name, email address, or mailing address changes. Keep your calendar up-to-date and accurate so you'll know when it's time to file important forms. Steps like these will help you protect yourself and your credit.

What Should I Do If I Cannot Pay?

Call your servicers immediately!

Financial difficulties happen — it's a fact of life. Your loan servicers know this, so if you have trouble making your loan payment, contact them.

Your servicers know all the options available to you and will help you devise a plan to successfully complete the repayment of your student loans.

Final Note

Don't forget the financial aid office staff at your institution. They are available to help you and are keenly aware of issues affecting medical students and graduates. Managing your loans can be a lot to sort through, so take it one step at a time.

Next Steps

The following is a brief guideline for soon-to-be graduates about the first steps for managing federal student loans as they transition into residency.

STEP 1 Immediately	**ORGANIZE YOUR LOANS** (refer to pages 6-8) • What types of loans do you have? • Who services the loans? • When is the first payment due?
STEP 2 30 Days Before Graduation	**HANDLE LOANS WITHOUT A GRACE PERIOD** (refer to pages 17-33) • Contact your servicers to request either a repayment plan or a forbearance to postpone payments. **CONSIDER PAYING SOME OF THE ACCRUED INTEREST** (refer to pages 14-16) • Check with the servicers to determine when your loans will capitalize.
STEP 3 Upon Graduation *(or Shortly After)*	**CONSOLIDATION IS AN OPTION** (refer to pages 59-63) • You can submit an application for immediate processing after your school reports you as separated, or you can request processing to begin at (or near) the end of the grace period. Consolidation processing takes 30-75 days; a consolidation can be initiated anytime after you're reported as no longer enrolled.
STEP 4 When Residency Begins	**IF YOU PLAN TO USE PSLF, COMPLETE A PSLF FORM** (refer to pages 55-58) • PSLF forms may be submitted now or anytime in the future.

STEP 5
Before the End of the Grace Period
	DECIDE IF YOU WILL POSTPONE OR BEGIN LOAN REPAYMENT (refer to pages 34-38)
	• 90 days before the end of the grace period, if you want to be in an income-driven repayment plan (ICR, IBR, PAYE, or REPAYE), you will submit your final application to the loan servicers (refer to pages 25-30).
	  ○ Earlier submissions will be denied even if you are eligible for the income-driven repayment plan selected.
	  ○ If you would prefer to make payments under the Standard, Extended, or Graduated Repayment plans, contact your loan servicers 30 days before the grace period expires or anytime thereafter.
	• 30 days before the end of the grace period, or anytime during residency, you are able to postpone payments with a Mandatory Medical Residency Forbearance (refer to pages 20-21).
	  ○ Contact your loan servicers to request this postponement option.

STEP 6 Before the End of the First Year	**SUBMIT RECERTIFICATION DOCUMENTS TO YOUR SERVICERS** • To continue in an income-driven repayment plan, submit documents about 90 days before the end of the first year of repayment. • To continue to postpone payments, reapply 30 days before the end of the first year of forbearance. • If pursuing PSLF, consider completing the PSLF form annually and immediately before and after any job change. • Repeat this step annually as appropriate.

Made in the USA
Middletown, DE
13 October 2022